At one moment this book is a heart-wrenching account of the devastating toll of Alzheimer's, and the next moment it is a heart-rending love story. The minute you are holding your breath at the brutality of the disease, Marty rescues you with a concrete, doable message that can lead to lovely moments of joy. No health care professional, family member, or caregiver should be without it.

— **Dawn Adler,** Director of Adult Day Center and ReCharge, Jewish Home and Care Center, Milwaukee; co-author of *Illuminate: An Integrated Curriculum for Early Memory Loss Programs*

My Two Elaines will touch the heart of every caregiver who has given his or her own to a loved one. Marty and Elaine Schreiber's journey together is at once unique and universal to so many. I served as a caregiver myself, for my grandmother, so I know the *mélange* of this experience. Marty shares his own experience in an honest and caring way. He walks us down a path that can be lonely, but *My Two Elaines* reminds us that caregivers are not alone. Marty's story of selflessness and struggle will offer strength for many caregivers across our country who act as everyday heroes.

— **U.S. Senator Tammy B**

My Two Elaines will no doubt offer caregivers of Alzheimer's patients some solace, practical insights, and a touch of humor as they daily face their daunting responsibilities. But for the primary care physicians, nurses, social workers, clergy, and others who support and care for these caregivers, Marty gives us an opportunity to see his world and better understand the grief and loss that is experienced and the very real physical and psychological manifestations that this stress creates. I encourage my fellow healthcare professionals to read and share this book. As we wait for the day that science eliminates this heart-wrenching disease, we can use the awareness gained to provide the empathy, care, and support that will allow these caregivers to continue this work of love.

— **Judy Beiler, RN**, Director, Global and Executive Health, Aurora Health Care, Milwaukee

If you or someone you know is a caregiver, this is a must-read. Your loved one really does become a different person. As I learned from my mom's dementia, learning how to deal with her was key to everyone's sanity. There are many helpful hints here.

— **Bonnie Blair**, five-time Olympic gold medalist

This book will resonate with caregivers and provides insight into the array of emotions and real-life challenges faced when caring for someone with Alzheimer's. The devastating impact of this disease is not lost in Marty's humor or endearing personal stories, but he offers solace in his lessons learned and how to appreciate what is left vs. what has been lost.

— **Kathy Cavers**, Administrator/COO,
The Lutheran Home, Milwaukee

Marty Schreiber has written a critically important book for Alzheimer's and dementia family caregivers. A natural storyteller, Marty blends wit, humor, and raw emotion into an immensely readable and compelling work. He does not hold back on the terrible toll Alzheimer's has taken on his and his family's life, but he also demonstrates for others that there is a path to eventual healing and survival. This book will not only help caregivers avoid some of the physical and emotional stresses they will inevitably face; it will also help them see their loved one with dementia in a new and better light as they navigate the Alzheimer's journey together.

— **Tom Hlavacek**, Executive Director, Alzheimer's Association Southeastern Wisconsin Chapter

My Two Elaines is the story of one man's experience with caring for his wife after her Alzheimer's diagnosis, but it's also one experienced by endless others. Personal and practical for anyone caring for a spouse or family member, Marty's writing directly addresses other men finding themselves in the role of husband-turned-caregiver. I only wish my father had this book to help him during my own mother's illness.

— **Paula Kiely**, City Librarian, Milwaukee Public Library

After working with seniors and in the health care field for over thirty years, I still continue to learn every day. This book has taught me many things, and I'm indebted to Marty.

— **Adele Lund**, Director, Community & Business Relations, Laureate Group senior housing communities, Milwaukee

This wonderful book gives a personal perspective of a couple's journey with Alzheimer's disease, as they reach out for help and support. The personal sharing, the compelling development of Marty, and his insight as a caregiver all provide for an important message.

— **Michael Malone, MD**, Medical Director, Aurora Health Care Senior Services; Chair, Public Policy Committee, American Geriatrics Society

Unfortunately, most of us will be affected by Alzheimer's in one manner or another over the course of our lives. Marty has truly captured the essence of loving and caring for somebody with this disease. His book is insightful, thoughtful, heartwarming, and respectful. Marty's sense of humor and abundant patience surely are a blessing for Elaine.

— **Scott McFadden**, President and CEO, The Lutheran Home & Harwood Place, Milwaukee

My Two Elaines demonstrates beautifully that the journey is not just for the person with the diagnosis but for the spouse and family as well and that it is a journey to not attempt alone and unsupported. The man-to-man discussions will no doubt help those who may be afraid to admit they don't have it all under control. I highly recommend this book. It is a quick read that provides a lot of great advice that will decrease the learning curve immensely.

— **Tara Reed**, author of *What to Do Between the Tears: A Practical Guide to Dealing with a Dementia or Alzheimer's Diagnosis in the Family*

My Two Elaines

*Learning, Coping, and Surviving
as an Alzheimer's Caregiver*

Martin J. Schreiber
with
Cathy Breitenbucher

BOOK PUBLISHERS NETWORK
Changing the World One Book at a Time

Book Publishers Network
P.O. Box 2256
Bothell • WA • 98041
Ph • 425-483-3040
www.bookpublishersnetwork.com

10 9 8 7 6 5 4 3 2 1

Printed in the United States of America

LCCN   2016954032
ISBN   978-1-945271-21-2

Names: Schreiber, Martin J., 1939- author. | Breitenbucher, Cathy, author.

Title: My two Elaines : learning, coping, and surviving as an Alzheimer's caregiver / by Martin J. Schreiber with Cathy Breitenbucher.

Description: Bothell, WA : Book Publishers Network, [2017] | Includes resources list.

Identifiers: ISBN: 978-1-945271-21-2 | LCCN: 2016954032

Subjects: LCSH: Schreiber, Elaine (Elaine Ruth Thaney), 1939- | Schreiber, Martin J., 1939- | Alzheimer's disease--Patients--Biography. | Alzheimer's disease--Patients--Home care. | Alzheimer's disease--Patients--Care. | Alzheimer's disease--Patients--Family relationships. | Alzheimer's disease--Patients--Services for. | Caregivers--United States--Biography. | Caregivers--United States--Handbooks, manuals, etc. | Caregivers--United States--Mental health. | Caregivers' writings, American. | Husband and wife. | LCGFT: Biographies. | Handbooks and manuals.

Classification: LCC: RC523 .S37 2017 | DDC: 362.1968/31--dc23

Editors: Amy Bauman, Julie Scandora
Cover Designers: Loni Theisen, Laura Zugzda
Photo Designer: Loni Theisen
Typographer: Andy Haas Schneider
Photo Restoration Assistant: Ange Bremeier

Net proceeds from the sales of *My Two Elaines* will be used to promote Alzheimer's caregiver support programs.

To my two Elaines

Contents

It wasn't until a few weeks ago that I really had to say, "Yes," I do have Alzheimer's. I had read of signs that indicate Alzheimer's, like getting overly upset for no reason and having trouble with names and directions. But I still didn't think it was a problem for me. But in hindsight . . . for too long, I've been getting lost driving, having trouble keeping days straight and difficulties with names and schedules. Still, I still felt I could handle it —"It won't get worse." But this morning, I started reading about the mid-stage of Alzheimer's, in hopes of preparing myself better, and realized I'm not very far away. That is most scary! But, I have to accept it.

— Elaine's letter to her "dear loved ones,"
dated March 11, 2009

Foreword

The names Martin and Elaine Schreiber will ring a bell for many in Wisconsin, especially political watchers. The story they know is that of the state's thirty-ninth governor and the first lady. Since 1962 when Martin won his first political race for state senate, they'd been familiar faces on the political circuit, crisscrossing the state in campaigns for lieutenant governor, then for governor. They made an elegant couple, greeting Bobby Kennedy, President Carter, and other national leaders when they came to Wisconsin. For almost thirty years, election night usually found the Schreibers side by side watching the returns come in for one of Marty's races, accepting the victories and the defeats with grace. Later, when his own political career had finished, Marty became one of the state's best-known government-relations consultants.

This was the story I knew in the beginning, the one familiar to so many, but it is not the one you will find in the pages of this book. *My Two Elaines* is instead the story of what happened to the Schreibers later in life when Elaine began to show the first signs of Alzheimer's disease and then gradually, but surely, came under its grip.

Although this is the Schreibers' personal tale, many Americans will recognize the broad outlines. Alzheimer's disease is now the sixth leading cause of death in the United States, claiming more than ninety-three thousand lives every year. And the numbers are bound to rise as modern medicine helps us to live longer. Alzheimer's is one of the great health challenges facing mankind in the twenty-first century. It is also a disease that inspires a unique kind of dread. We find it terrifying to imagine a time when the body will continue to function but the mind will slip away.

So, in practical terms, *My Two Elaines* is an invaluable guide to millions who will face Alzheimer's in the role of patient or caregiver. In its pages, you will find a knowing and sympathetic guide to the day-to-day work of living with the disease. And it's important you have no illusions, for work it is.

Marty is clear about that.

When I first got to know the former governor in 2015 in the course of writing a story on loneliness, I was struck by his honesty. Politicians are gregarious, but on their own terms. They spend so much of their time letting us see only the good qualities, the strong ones. On the campaign circuit, vulnerability may not count for much, but in everyday life, it is deeply underrated. It is the quality that infuses *My Two Elaines* with its power and makes it a valuable addition to the literature on Alzheimer's. To his great credit, Marty opens his life fully as a husband and Alzheimer's caregiver. He allows readers to see the sorrow, the frustration, even the anger that comes from watching this disease destroy someone you love. He also describes the small moments of joy that even Alzheimer's cannot take away.

But it would not do justice to the book to file it away among the how-to or self-help guides. I read and enjoyed *My Two Elaines* most of all as a love story. The Schreibers' love for each other shines through on every page. It endures the worst insults that Alzheimer's heaps upon the living. It endures even as the disease constructs a wall between the couple and the rich years they've shared.

In its raw honesty, the book itself is an act of love. Stories make us feel less alone in the world. Marty has generously given us his and Elaine's.

— **Mark Johnson,** Pulitzer Prize winner and co-author of *One in a Billion: The Story of Nic Volker and the Dawn of Genomic Medicine*

Preface

I felt compelled to write this book in the hope that relating my experience in caring for my wife with Alzheimer's disease would help other caregivers learn, cope, and survive. While sharing this message man-to-man was a primary objective, those who looked over the manuscript told me they believed this book could help a wider audience as well. So, I invite families and friends to use it to better understand Alzheimer's, learn how to assist the caregiver, and help the patient experience moments of joy even as they daily face the overwhelming sadness of this disease. In addition, I am told my story may resonate with women who are caregivers; therefore, you'll see references to *partner*, *spouse*, or *loved one*.

Because I believe that maintaining a sense of humor is helping me bear up under the stress of Alzheimer's, I have included some anecdotes at the beginning of several chapters that I hope make you laugh. If my icebreakers aren't your style, I beg your forgiveness as you focus on the book's central messages.

It wasn't until I was almost finished with the manuscript that I began finding many diaries, notes, and letters that Elaine had written at various times after her diagnosis. These writings sparked sadness in realizing at times I hadn't been able to be a better caregiver, and yet they also brought joy to know that I'd made her feel happy and comforted. Until I read Elaine's own words, I never had a full comprehension of her emotions: her fears and anxieties, her love, and ultimately her courage. I am so pleased I can share a fuller picture of Elaine by including her side of the story, too.

Unless otherwise stated, statistics cited here are from the Alzheimer's Association, which since 1980 has led the world in Alzheimer's care, support, and research. For information and support, call the Alzheimer's Association twenty-four-hour helpline (1-800-272-3900) or visit alz.org.

Introduction

I met my First Elaine as a freshman at Milwaukee Lutheran High School in 1953. My last name—Schreiber—and hers—Thaney—put us pretty close in classroom seating.

My First Elaine helped me achieve each one of my successes and stood by me in every one of my losses and illnesses. She helped me pass biology at the University of Wisconsin-Milwaukee (remember alphabetical seating, mentioned above). She worked as a secretary to put me through Marquette University Law School. She pushed our daughter, Kathy, in a stroller while campaigning door-to-door for my first race in 1962; when I won, she won, too. She celebrated with me later that year when I was elected to the Wisconsin State Senate. Four years later and pregnant, she kept four-year-old Kathy and our son Marty, age three, neat and presentable during a station-wagon tour of all seventy-two counties in Wisconsin in my race for lieutenant governor. I lost and continued to serve in the state senate.

I did win election as lieutenant governor in 1970, and eventually we had four children. In 1977, I became the thirty-ninth governor of Wisconsin. There were more campaigns to run—for governor in 1978 and 1982 and mayor of Milwaukee in 1988. I lost those, too, but I was experienced at not always coming out on top. As I've said many times in my life, my role in law school was to assure that there would be an upper 50 percent of the graduating class. Elaine uncomplainingly went to work as a teacher to get our family back on stable financial ground after my political run ended. I am profoundly grateful for her support.

We may have lost elections, but she never let me be defeated. In my second career, I've worked in insurance, publishing, and government affairs. The high of being a husband, a father, a grandfather, and now a great-grandfather surpasses any thrill I ever experienced in politics or business.

Elaine was as intelligent, kind, gracious, loving, understanding, self-sacrificing, and forgiving as any wife, mother, or grandmother could ever be. She was a perfect wife—she cooked, kept house, raised the children, held dinner parties, dressed stylishly, took me to chemotherapy as I battled cancer, and sailed with me.

If it weren't for her, there wouldn't be me.

Starting in about 2005, that Elaine began to slip away from me. Her daily skills declined, and her interest in long-held hobbies withered. The time came when she could not drive without getting lost. Over time, my constant helpmate became dependent on me for everything. Today, she does not cook, keep house, hold dinner parties, or dress herself. She forgot her grandchildren and got lost on our boat and in our home of twenty years.

Even with Alzheimer's disease, Elaine remains as kind, gracious, loving, and self-sacrificing as any person could be. But she is not the same person. My First Elaine gave way to my Second Elaine.

I have hoped, laughed, and cried with both of them, just as you have with your wife or husband—and I now have had to acknowledge that the future will not unfold the way I thought it would.

With my First Elaine, we shared love, hope, happiness, and dreams. As my First Elaine became my Second, the dreams turned into nightmares because I was losing her. Happiness became hopelessness. Grieving and health issues (including depression and anxiety) replaced joy.

I greatly miss my First Elaine. My heart broke as she left me. It was so painful as this "new normal" enveloped us with Alzheimer's destroying the memories we had created over decades. I still love her, of course, but in a quite different way. I still want to make her happy, even when she is confused, unsettled, anxious, and much less aware of most things in life.

One day about five years into her disease, the Second Elaine asked me how we got together.

"Well," I told her, "when you were fourteen, I saw how pretty and smart and nice you were. I determined I wanted you for my wife, and if any other boys got within fifty feet of you, I bopped them on the head."

"You're a bullshitter," she said. My First Elaine would never have used language like that! When it came out, it was a bit shocking but funny, so I laughed, and she laughed. The new Elaine was speaking out. We shared an unexpected moment of joy.

"Well," I said, "let's just keep that between you and me."

"Oh no," she insisted. "It won't do any good. Everyone already knows."

* * *

It is said that there are more books written about Abraham Lincoln than any other subject in American nonfiction. When your spouse has dementia, you might feel that our sixteenth president has given way to Dr. Alois Alzheimer, the German physician who pioneered the study of memory loss. Before you became an Alzheimer's caregiver, you never dreamed there was so much material out there—medical journals, memoirs, poetry, essays, and more. Sadly, with 5.2

million Americans age sixty-five and older currently diagnosed with Alzheimer's and 7.1 million expected to be challenged by the disease by the year 2025, it's a growth industry.

Over the course of my wife's ten-year struggle with Alzheimer's, I've looked at plenty of those books. I didn't benefit much from the bookish science stuff or the bullet-point how-tos. Not one of the books I read conveyed the ugly truth about caregiving: that it can destroy you—even kill you—if you go about it wrong. I hope this book speaks to you so that you can help your partner on his or her Alzheimer's journey be the best caregiver possible, and survive.

What I have learned over the past decade will, I hope, make a difference in your life and that of your loved one. I have hiked up the Alzheimer's mountain, have identified its dangerous areas, and am meeting you now on the way back down, as you begin your own climb. Please, don't take another step until you hear what I have to say.

As you know—unfortunately, tragically—you are at a moment when it is impossible for you to avoid taking this journey. You are unable to turn back. Your health, your spirit, your very life all are in danger unless you learn more about what lies ahead. By knowing where the hazards are, you can avoid some of the mistakes I have made and, in doing so, better help your spouse deal with this disease.

One in nine older people in the United States currently has Alzheimer's. Statistically speaking, it is a woman's disease—almost two-thirds of Americans with Alzheimer's are female. That's 3.3 million individual tragedies, as of 2015. Yet, when you find out that your partner has Alzheimer's, you feel utterly alone. You used to share your problems with and get support from this person, but now you can't. Your partner is no longer your partner; he or she is your responsibility. Suddenly, you don't know where to turn. So, you dig in your heels, convinced that you can outlast this disease. Especially if you're the man of the household, you may feel you have a tough-guy image to maintain. You worked hard, raised a family, built a business or two . . . or maybe even governed a state.

For men who are caregivers, the definition of manhood changes when their wife has Alzheimer's. It's not about being tough; it's about being smart. It's going to be hard for you to change your thinking, I know. The real way to demonstrate your manhood—and I learned this the hard way—is to not try to go it alone. Asking for help does not mean you're less of a man.

This advice applies to female caregivers as well. Wives are used to doing it all—juggling the family's schedules, keeping the house in order, doing the bulk of shopping and meal preparation, and often working outside the home, too. Taking care of someone with dementia makes a sizable dent in the time and energy available for those other necessary tasks. Asking for help does not mean you're less of a wife.

Let me be your trail guide. I will tell you why it's essential to reach out for help. Many of these thoughts will be found throughout the book on sticky notes titled "What I wish I'd known." I can show you how to cope in notes labeled "What I wish I'd done."

I'll also try to teach you how allowing yourself moments of joy can help you survive. And I'll do it with a little humor. Without humor, you'll go nuts.

While on your journey, your beloved partner will be replaced by someone with the same name in the same body. Your loved one's mind will be even more different than you can imagine. As time passes, his or her memory will be erased to such a degree that most of the memories of your life together are partially missing or completely gone. You will experience someone behaving and talking in a manner completely different from the person you have known and loved. Can there be anything more painful? Probably not. I call it death by a thousand cuts. But know this: there are Band-Aids for these cuts—resources and help of which you must take advantage.

As a caregiver, you will do heroic work. You're thinking: "Me? A hero?" I say, "Yes! A hero!" Even though your efforts will not be enough to stop the disease from stealing your partner away from you, the deeds you will perform are heroic as you continue to care for and love your partner.

No job or responsibility you've ever shouldered will be as challenging as this new role. When your partner has Alzheimer's, almost without thinking, you will put his or her needs above yours. Eventually you realize you've gone from 100 percent spouse to 100 percent caregiver. Your skills and patience will be tested to the point where you think you too are losing your mind. Being a caregiver to someone who no longer knows your name would have been the last thing you thought of on that long-ago wedding day when you vowed to take your loved one "in sickness and in health." But here you are. It hurts, and it takes its toll, more so when you don't get help.

No one gets to be a hero without being prepared. Not the D-Day invasion force, not the Apollo 13 crew, not even the local high school quarterback. Starting right now, you must step aside from all the busyness to understand yourself as a caregiver-hero. The sooner you focus on your new role truthfully, the better you can cope. You owe it to yourself and to your loved one to get this right. In the end, all you can say is that you did your best. That makes you a hero.

My heart goes out to you. But remember: learn about Alzheimer's, learn how to cope with it, learn how to survive.

Learning about Alzheimer's Disease

I'm so lucky he is a good cook and seems to enjoy making healthy and delicious meals. It's a good thing as my Alzheimer's isn't getting any better, so cooking and baking with steps that need to work are no longer easy for me. I hate to think I am getting worse, but I must be

— Elaine's Florida journal,
dated March 31, 2012

—CHAPTER 1—
Diagnosis

My first experience with Alzheimer's was in 1978 when I was campaigning for governor. One bright fall day, I was giving a speech in Eau Claire, a college town in northwestern Wisconsin. It was essentially the same stump speech I'd been using all over the state to warm applause. Afterward, I was shaking some hands when an elderly gentleman came up to me. "That was the worst god-awful speech I ever heard," he snarled.

His wife followed behind quickly, wearing an embarrassed look. She apologized several times. "Governor, you've got to understand," she pleaded. "He's old and senile, and all he ever does is repeat whatever he hears everyone else say."

* * *

When you learn that your loved one has Alzheimer's disease, it's the beginning of the end. It's easy to say that the diagnosis marks both an end and a beginning, and to a degree that's true. There's a "before" and an "after" to this news. But one part of your life doesn't instantly come to an end while another part magically crops up to take its place.

Dementia is a general term for a decline in mental ability severe enough to interfere with daily life. Not every dementia is Alzheimer's; however, some forms of dementia, such as dementia with Lewy bodies and Creutzfeldt-Jakob disease, are equally devastating and fatal diseases. Some people have what's called mixed dementia—the combination of Alzheimer's and another type of dementia.

On the other hand, people can have temporary symptoms of dementia after a stroke or because of medical conditions, including depression, urinary tract infections, thyroid problems, and vitamin deficiencies, or adverse drug reactions. Issues such as these often can be successfully treated. So, if a loved one is confused and anxious, don't panic and think the worst. ***Have a doctor check for all possible explanations.***

Alzheimer's, however, is the best-known, most common form of dementia. It accounts for 60 percent to 80 percent of all dementia cases. It is unrelenting and irreversible, and it can drag on for years before it kills someone you love dearly. There. I just said what we all fear the most. This time around, I'm not being a BSer.

For those with dementia, the most fearful time may be that period when they know they are losing their mind and worry what the future outcome will be. It's a horrible thing to witness. One of the worst episodes in Elaine's and my realization that there was a problem was when she was preparing one of her favorite German meals for several friends who had come to our home for dinner. Although she'd been using these recipes for years, she got all mixed up and left out some of the ingredients. The food was inedible. But far worse was the desperate and sad look on Elaine's face as she understood why this was happening.

When something like that occurs, instinctively you help your partner more, or you start ordering pizza every night. Instead of addressing what is really going on, you just adapt. You sort of get used to it—and that's a form of denial. Months pass, and maybe you mention it to the doctor.

By the time you go to an Alzheimer's specialist, you have a pretty good sense of what's happening with your partner. Why else would you have made that appointment?

A diagnosis of Alzheimer's presents a real ethical challenge for doctors and caregivers. Is it better for the patient to know or to not know? It's a topic of such importance that the Alzheimer's Association issued a ten-page Special Report in its 2015 Alzheimer's Disease Facts and Figures book. Studies cited in the report found that only 45 percent of people with Alzheimer's and their family members reported ever being told of the diagnosis. Experts say there are benefits to knowing. These include having the time to make financial plans and the opportunity to be educated about and have access to support services.

For us, the news wasn't a big shock, based on the symptoms Elaine had been showing. As far back as 2005, when Elaine was sixty-five years old, she told a psychiatrist that she'd had concerns about her memory for a couple of years already. She explained that she sometimes had difficulty driving; when she got confused, she needed to stop the car to regain her sense of direction. Cognitive tests revealed a mixed bag: some memory skills were ranked as "average" and some "low average." None of those scores were in the "impaired" range.

In 2007, the doctor began to dig deeper. For one thing, he ordered an MRI of the brain. The scan didn't particularly point to trouble; in fact, it ruled out the possibility that Elaine had had a stroke. But her behavior was telling us that her brain was changing. Doctor appointments became more frequent.

At one appointment, she mentioned that she was having trouble remembering what she'd read, whether it was in newspapers or novels. She had all but given up on reading. At another appointment, she was able to easily give the receptionist her date of birth, but five minutes later in the exam room, she couldn't come up with it at all. At that point, she was given a different cognitive test called the Mini-Mental State Examination (MMSE). It was similar to the assessment she'd been given before: repeat a short list of words, name what month it is, draw the face of a clock—that kind of thing. The scoring tops out at thirty, with people in the thirty to twenty-eight range considered to have normal cognitive ability, twenty-seven to twenty-five possible mild cognitive impairment, and so on down the line. Elaine scored a twenty-eight.

People with Alzheimer's can and do function well in the early stages of the disease. Just because you were diagnosed on Tuesday doesn't mean you can't put together a perfectly good sandwich or spreadsheet on Thursday. A year or two from Thursday? That's another matter.

As for Elaine, at the time of her diagnosis, she still took care of her basic needs, managed the house and was socially engaged. On the surface, she was still the gracious First Lady of Wisconsin who had welcomed artists, championship sports teams, Lillian Carter, and even the crown princess of Norway to the Executive Residence. If you didn't ask how long she'd stay at a twenty-eight or how she'd behave when she'd be at a twenty-two, it lulled you into thinking, *This isn't so bad.*

What I wish I'd known

A person with Alzheimer's will experience diminished mental capabilities at a rate of three to five points per year on the MMSE scale. But, it doesn't happen in a predictable way.

Still, the diagnosis was a milestone event: it came with her first prescription for an Alzheimer's drug—Aricept (donepezil). It's an oral medication that works to temporarily alter the brain chemistry so that nerve cells can continue to trade information with one another. The doctor also recommended that she have a neurological evaluation.

Later that year, soon after Elaine turned sixty-eight, I sought out the best neurologist I could find, at the Medical College of Wisconsin in Milwaukee. The examination and tests only confirmed what we had been told before.

Alzheimer's.

Beyond that, I honestly don't remember what words the doctor used. I'm sure he didn't say, "There is no hope" or "This is fatal." I already knew the one absolute about Alzheimer's: no one survives it. I do recall him emphasizing the importance of socialization, Aricept and another drug called Namenda (memantine) to temporarily improve symptoms, plus daily exercise and a glass of red wine every night. Jokingly, I said that Elaine was two weeks behind on the exercise and two months ahead on the red wine.

We didn't need a third opinion. I respected the doctors we had. We left the clinic clinging to the notion that we could set our own course and somehow slow down the Alzheimer's death march. Like the good teacher she was (and in spite of her current difficulties with reading), Elaine headed to the library for every Alzheimer's book she could get her hands on. She devoured them, taking note after note almost as if she could beat the disease based on the number of books she read and notes she made. It also seemed that she was doing some type of penance or seeking forgiveness for the problems she knew she would later cause.

Deep down, she knew how bad it was going to get. She was dealing with the painful realization that she was going to lose her memory, her independence, her dignity, and eventually her life. Out loud, she worried that she would be abandoned. Would I still love her? Would I still take care of her?

"When I get to be a burden," she'd say, "you can put me away."

Many nights, we cried ourselves to sleep.

* * *

Scientists have been studying memory loss for better than a hundred years. In 1906, Alois Alzheimer first lectured on "an unusual disease of the cerebral cortex" that he had observed. Ever since—particularly since 1980, when the Alzheimer's Association was founded—some of the brightest minds in medicine have worked to unravel this terrible disease.

Tremendous progress has been made over the past generation in treating many other diseases. Childhood cancer is a great example. The American Cancer Society says the overall five-year survival rate has climbed from about 58 percent in the mid-1970s to more than 80 percent today.

But when it comes to Alzheimer's, we're hardly better off today than we were a hundred years ago. Most babies who were born in Alois Alzheimer's time didn't live past the age of fifty, according to the National Institute on Aging. Meanwhile, babies born in the United States today are projected to live to just under seventy-nine years of age, according to Centers for Disease Control and Prevention. That longer lifespan gives Alzheimer's more of an opportunity to develop. And then there are the baby boomers, reaching age sixty-five at the rate of about ten thousand a day—a figure estimated to continue until the year 2030. So the race is on to find a cure.

It takes years for any drug—such as those that blessedly have improved childhood cancer survival—to be approved for use in the United States by the Food and Drug Administration (FDA). Contrary to what you might think, the FDA itself does not develop drugs. That happens in universities, hospitals, and pharmaceutical labs all over the world. For those of us without a scientific mind, the process seems ridiculously tedious: develop a theory, design a way to test it, run into a dead end, re-examine the theory, design a new test, run into a dead end, etc., etc., etc. until you hit on something.

Once there are promising data from lab studies, drug developers have to submit what's called an Investigational New Drug (IND) application to the FDA's Center for Drug Evaluation and Research (CDER). CDER's mission is to ensure that drugs marketed in this country are safe and effective. CDER does not test drugs, although it has an Office of Testing and Research that conducts limited research in the areas of drug quality, safety, and effectiveness. And I thought state government was a bureaucracy!

Only after an IND application is approved can the drug's sponsor begin testing on humans. Clinical trials are funded by pharmaceutical companies and medical device manufacturers, academic medical centers, foundations or individuals, organizations such as the Alzheimer's Association, or governmental agencies.

According to the National Institutes of Health, there are four phases to a clinical trial:

Phase I: Researchers test the drug or treatment in a small group of people for the first time to evaluate its safety, determine a safe dosage range, and identify side effects.

Phase II: The drug or treatment is given to a larger group of people to see if it is effective and to further evaluate its safety.

Phase III: The drug or treatment is given to large groups of people to confirm its effectiveness, monitor side effects, compare it to commonly used treatments, and collect information that will allow the drug or treatment to be used safely.

Phase IV: Studies are done after the drug or treatment has been marketed to gather information on the drug's effect in various populations and any side effects associated with long-term use.

Sometimes, a drug doesn't even make it through all the phases of a clinical trial. End of story. Back to the drawing board.

From 2002 to 2012, a total of 244 Alzheimer's drugs were tested with exactly one successfully completing the trials process and being approved by the FDA. One!

So far, the drugs that have been approved by the FDA for use in treating Alzheimer's only slow the worsening of *symptoms* of the disease. They are effective for about six to twelve months, on average, for about half of the individuals who take them. Unfortunately, they don't treat the underlying disease or delay its progression. And only five such drugs are in use. That includes one that got the OK in 2014, which was a combination of two previously approved drugs. Before that, the last time an Alzheimer's drug was approved for use in the United States was in 2003.

So there you have it. The cold, hard truth is that despite the gallant efforts of scientists around the world, there currently is no cure or even a decent way to slow down the brain-damaging effects of Alzheimer's. When your partner is diagnosed, you don't do yourself any favors by sticking your head in the sand. I hate to tell you, but it's going to get worse. It just is.

Alzheimer's doesn't stand still. Your partner will become someone you don't know. And you will become someone you don't recognize: a caregiver. At first, you don't call yourself that. You're simply a spouse who is caring for a loved one who is confused. But then without realizing it, and with no ability to stop this transformation, you morph from being a full-time partner into a full-time caregiver.

What I wish I'd done

Right away, I should have taken full advantage of all that the Alzheimer's Association has to offer. Besides support groups, there is individual counseling— plus online tools and information.

Sometimes, a person's decline is the steady, annoying but non-emergency drip-drip-drip of the bathroom faucet at 3:00 a.m. At other times, it's as if you're filling the watering can for the garden, you turn your back for just a moment, and when you look again, the water is overflowing the can and creating a muddy mess. Big declines can sometimes occur if there are additional medical issues, such as a urinary tract infection.

We're a nation of doers. We aim high, and we despise failure. We keep score on the sports field and in the political arena. We look at a problem—such as that drippy bathroom faucet—and we figure it out. Alzheimer's can't be fixed, not yet anyway. But, take heart; there is help available so you can meet the challenge of life as a caregiver.

About three years after Elaine's diagnosis, one of the nurses at the neurologist's office asked me whether

I'd joined any support groups. Who, me? I'm from that generation of men who weren't supposed to even have feelings, much less show them in public. Does the name Edmund Muskie ring a bell? He was a fine US senator from Maine, a leading candidate for the Democratic presidential nomination in 1972. But his bid fell apart on a snowy New Hampshire morning when he denounced a newspaper story that was critical of his wife. Of all things, the article noted that his wife liked to enjoy a drink before dinner, tell bawdy jokes, and smoke cigarettes. Some reports asserted that Muskie cried as he defended his wife, while others said he merely choked up. Either way, opponents used the incident to claim Muskie was too emotional to run the country. He withdrew from the race not long after.

As for me, I was not man enough to know I needed help to deal with my wife's health problem. My feeling was I didn't need a pity party. The problem with that attitude was that I didn't know what Alzheimer's support groups were all about—I wrongly thought I'd be sitting in a circle of weepy people telling "can you top this?" stories about their loved one's behaviors.

I was doing fine (I thought). I'd be OK (I thought).

But as they say, pride goeth before the fall.

My Marty, who is and always has been my strength and comfort. I thank God every day for his understanding, loving ways, patience, good humor, hard work. He has made possible not only four wonderful children and a wonderfully exciting and busy life for me, but also helped so many others throughout his lifetime. He has a true gift for making those around him feel good about themselves, laugh at his jokes, and grow into stronger people. I thank you for that, Hon, as I've benefitted the most.

— Elaine's letter to her "dear loved ones," dated March 11, 2009

—CHAPTER 2—
When Marty Met Elaine

If you believe in love at first sight, then I fell in love with Elaine Ruth Thaney in the fall of 1953. We were freshmen in Latin class at Milwaukee Lutheran High School (MLHS), which was located at Thirteenth and Vine Streets, just west of where Interstate 43 now makes its way from downtown to the North Shore suburbs. In those post-war years, enrollment was growing so quickly that the school building, constructed in 1908, was bursting at the seams. Old army barracks were added to the property to provide enough classroom space. It didn't matter that there were hundreds of girls at MLHS; I knew right away Elaine was the one for me. Apparently she thought so, too, because we didn't date anyone else through high school.

At the start of our junior year, MLHS moved to a newly constructed building in a sparsely populated area on the northwest side of Milwaukee. That same year, Disneyland opened in California, Jonas Salk's polio vaccine was declared safe and effective, and in Montgomery, Alabama, Rosa Parks refused to give up her seat on the bus to a white passenger. Change was everywhere, except when it came to Elaine and me. We were in love.

I was raised on Center Street near North Twenty-Fifth Street in a small house behind my father's real estate office. He had served a term in the state assembly and later was elected to Milwaukee's city council. Our house featured just one bedroom, so my father, who was well-trained as a carpenter, put partitions in the attic to create bedrooms for me, my older sister, and my kid brother.

Elaine grew up on Grant Boulevard in the Sherman Park area, which is still a desirable neighborhood in Milwaukee because of its beautiful brick and quarried-stone homes. The first time I drove her there, I saw these magnificent residences, and I couldn't believe how big they were. *Wow,* I thought to myself. Then she said, "My house is on the other side of the street," and it was a very modest structure. There went any delusions I had about marrying for money! Her father owned a company that made concrete blocks. He worked very hard to keep the business going so he could support his family. He would tell Elaine, "God made me rich with five children."

Elaine was the oldest child. A bright girl, she was one of those kids you loved to hate because it seemed she always got As and never needed to study. But she had well-rounded interests—she was selected as a cheerleader, was a member of the synchronized swimming team, and even took up the drums. She later told me she did that so she could be with me in the school band; it didn't hurt that a set of drumsticks cost maybe seventy-five cents, well within her family's budget. I played second chair clarinet.

It was rare that I outshone Elaine. When I was elected as a class officer, it was largely because she helped by painting clever red and blue campaign signs that looked like "wanted" posters.

Elaine's generous spirit was evident throughout her teenage years. When I turned sixteen, she took up a collection from our friends to rent a park pavilion for a surprise birthday party. From the money our classmates chipped in, she proudly presented me with water skis that cost eighteen dollars—quite a sum in the mid-1950s. When she turned sixteen a few months later, she got her first real job, at a dry cleaning business managed by an elderly woman. Knowing that this lady had no relatives, Elaine insisted one year that we buy a small Christmas tree and take it to her.

After high school, Elaine headed to Concordia, a Lutheran college in River Forest, Illinois, to study to be a teacher. I wanted to be either an attorney or a minister, and I went to a different Lutheran school,

Valparaiso University, in northwestern Indiana. By car, our colleges were about an hour and a half apart. Long-distance phone calls cost something like $1.75 for three minutes, which was never long enough for me. I was worried I might lose her to a boy at Concordia.

With money tight in her family, Elaine transferred after her freshman year to a public school, the University of Wisconsin's main campus in Madison. I had given up any aspirations I had to become a minister, so I left Valparaiso University to enroll at the University of Wisconsin-Milwaukee. We were back in the same state again, but still an hour and a half apart. After a year in Madison, Elaine decided to join me at UW-Milwaukee. That was my saving grace, personally and academically. Without Elaine sitting next to me in botany and biology, I never could have passed those classes. She had a keen mind in the classroom.

But Elaine put her education on hold for me. After our junior year of college, I was accepted into a program across town at Marquette University that gave me a jump-start on law school. Elaine took a full-time job as a secretary (and I worked construction over the summers) to save money so we could get married, which we did on June 3, 1961. I had two years of law school remaining.

They say timing is everything, and I lucked out in the spring of 1962. My parents had recently co-signed the mortgage for a seventy-five-hundred-dollar duplex near North Twenty-Fifth and Monroe Streets. Then a vacancy occurred in the state senate, in the very district where we lived, giving me the opportunity to run for office. One of my opponents in the four-man primary was Fred Kessler, who, believe it or not, had been a high school classmate of ours at Milwaukee Lutheran. He had been elected to the state assembly in 1960 at the age of twenty.

My dad was serving as a Milwaukee alderman, so I benefitted from his name recognition with the voters. But my real advantage in the primary was Elaine. She took it upon herself to go downtown to the election commission office for the names of the newly registered voters, of which there were hundreds. Then, she used maps and lists of polling places to write postcards to tell each new voter exactly where to vote. I have fond memories of Elaine's enthusiasm as she sat on our living room floor, surrounded by piles of postcards that needed to be hand-addressed and personalized. I considered it rather risky because—let's face it—mistakes could be made or a person might just vote for the other candidate! She proved to be an astute campaign worker as I squeaked past Fred by 350 votes—a victory at age twenty-three that charted our whole life. Two months later in the general election, I received 76 percent of the vote.

No time to celebrate, though. I was still wrapping up law school. After I took my oath of office in January 1963, I attended the Tuesday through Thursday legislative sessions, which meant two nights a week in Madison. Elaine had her hands full with our young daughter, Kathy, and we were expecting again—our son Marty was born in April 1963. In 1964, I faced only token opposition in the general election.

Our third child was on the way in 1966 when I was running for lieutenant governor. The job paid $7,500 a year, compared to the $8,900 salary of a state senator. Elaine didn't bat an eye over that potential pay cut; she knew my goal was to become governor. It was obvious she was willing to do anything for me, including encouraging me to plan campaign events for late September, despite that being when our baby was due. I had early-morning plant gate appearances scheduled for September 28 in Beloit, about an hour southwest of Milwaukee, with plans to be home by early afternoon. Before I left home at 4:30 a.m., I asked Elaine if she was OK, and she assured me she was.

"I'm fine," she replied. "You go."

Around 10:00 a.m., though, our daughter Kristine was ready to enter our hectic world. Elaine walked herself to the nearby St. Joseph Hospital—where she herself had been born in 1939—and soon I got a call at the library where I was speaking to tell me that our baby daughter had arrived.

I lost that election and went back to the state senate, biding my time for another shot in 1970. By then, the state constitution had been changed so that the candidates for lieutenant governor and governor ran together. So, running in 1970 with Patrick Lucey at the top of the ticket, we were elected. One newspaper article described me as the Lucey ticket putting its best foot forward. Elaine was so proud and excited for me. She made our daughters' dresses and her own for the inauguration. In 1974, the Lucey-Schreiber team won re-election. Our family celebrated again in 1975 when our son Matt was born.

In case you don't remember the 1976 presidential election, Jimmy Carter narrowly defeated the Republican incumbent, Gerald R. Ford. That meant Carter could, among other things, pick a new ambassador to Mexico. Carter nominated his fellow Democrat, Patrick Lucey, and after Lucey was confirmed by the United States Senate, I succeeded him as governor on July 6, 1977. We held an open house at the Executive Residence the next day—7/7/77—and, despite a hot summer sun, the line stretched down the driveway and out into the street. We shook thousands of hands!

The 1970s were a roller coaster of a decade for us with my campaigning all over the state and my duties in Madison. At one point, we had a teenager, a baby and two kids in between. How Elaine held it all together and made it look so effortless is beyond me. Did I mention that she also went back to college and completed her education degree in 1974?

As a kid, I had prayed that I'd someday be governor. Maybe I should have prayed for five four-year terms—I mean, why not go for it?—because my time in office proved to be much shorter than I had hoped. In the 1978 election, a political newcomer named Lee S. Dreyfus ran an unconventional campaign and beat me with about 55 percent of the vote. My, could he orate! I moved on to an executive position at Sentry Insurance in Stevens Point in central Wisconsin, and we bought a forty-four-acre hobby farm in the next county over. Our daughter Kathy stayed in Madison to finish high school, but our three younger children moved with us and enjoyed the slower pace of country living. We had animals galore. When our goat gave birth to triplet kids (a somewhat rare event), we named them "Breakfast," "Lunch," and "Dinner." Meanwhile, Elaine and her friend Barbara opened an antiques and crafts store in the farm's restored granary building. Although it barely broke even, she enjoyed it.

Elaine was upbeat and positive in every campaign. She always told me, "Don't be afraid of losing." I guess that was good advice because I didn't make it out of the primary in the 1982 gubernatorial election. A couple of years later, we headed home to Milwaukee, where I hoped to be elected mayor in 1988, but I fell short in the general election. The major rap against me, as I recall, was that I was too nice to be mayor.

Over the next few years, we worked hard to relaunch our careers—Elaine as a teacher and I as a public-affairs consultant. Elaine even went back to college and earned a master's of education when she was fifty-six years old. She gave her heart to the at-risk preschoolers at the Silver Spring Neighborhood Center on Milwaukee's northwest side, and later led a successful capital campaign to benefit that organization. Because of her devotion, Silver Spring named its early-childhood development center for Elaine, an honor that was read into the Congressional Record by United States Representative Gwendolyn Moore.

At the same time, the kids grew up and moved out. Having married so young, we were empty nesters by our early fifties. We found fulfillment as volunteers and board members for organizations around town. Such good times!

We thought it would last forever.

I'd be so lost without you—so please continue to take good care of yourself for me as well as for you.

— A note from Elaine to Marty in 2013

CHAPTER 3

Danger on the Trail: How Alzheimer's Can Harm *Your* Health

Ever hear the one about the hippopotamus and the butterfly who fell in love? As the hippo begins thinking about proposing and consummating the marriage, he quickly realizes he has a problem. So, he seeks out the wise old owl for advice.

The owl says, "I can see that this is troubling you. You've come to the wisest animal for advice. Here's your answer: what you've got to do is turn yourself into a butterfly."

The hippo starts to walk away but quickly realizes that he doesn't know just how he can do that. He returns to Mr. Owl and says, "I would do anything for my dear loved one. Please tell me, how can I change myself into a butterfly?"

"Sorry, buster," the owl replies. "I just determine policy."

* * *

Like that owl, no matter how wise you think you are, Alzheimer's has truths about it that you cannot change. Your spouse is going to get worse, mentally and physically. No one's got the answer to that. And you're likely to suffer mental and physical harm, too. That shouldn't come as a big shocker because caregiving is a continuous process that puts unprecedented demands on your time, energy, and emotions. You cannot afford to be as arrogant as that owl.

If it makes you feel any better, you are not alone. It is estimated that, in 2015, there were 15.9 million Americans providing unpaid care for people with Alzheimer's and other forms of dementia. If you think 15.9 million sounds like a lot of people, you're right. It's eleven times the US workforce of Walmart!

All those tasks you take on—out of love, concern, and a sense of responsibility—add up to an average of almost twenty-two hours per week. So, nationwide caregivers provided 18.1 billion hours of unpaid assistance in 2015. That's billion with a *b*.

Here's another way of looking at what caregivers do. The federal minimum wage is $7.25 an hour. Paid home health aides' salaries average $17.24 an hour, reports the US Department of Labor. The care you are providing has to be worth more than what a fast-food worker makes, right? But maybe it's not as valuable as that of a trained professional health aide. So average those two salaries, and it's $12.25 an hour. Of course, you're not in it for the money. But if all of us caregivers banded together, we'd have given $221.3 billion worth of care in 2015.

Caregiving for people with dementia cuts across every demographic group you can think of. It is the job of the well-educated (more than 40 percent have at least a college degree), as well as those with modest incomes (41 percent have a household income of fifty thousand dollars or less).

One-third of Alzheimer's caregivers are, like me, over the age of sixty-five. But some caregivers are young children. A 2005 study by the National Alliance for Caregiving found that 250,000 kids in this country between the ages of eight and eighteen provide help to persons with Alzheimer's or another form of dementia.

As you become an Alzheimer's caregiver, you do so without the benefit of training. Those professional home health aides I mentioned a minute ago? Federal regulations require seventy-five hours of training to get a job with a Medicare-certified home health agency, according to the Paraprofessional Healthcare Institute. (In my home state of Wisconsin, it's 120 hours). For family caregivers, though, it's learning on the job, a baptism by fire.

Being an Alzheimer's caregiver takes a tremendous toll, but it happens in such a gradual way that you may not notice how harmful it is to you. Exercise? Eat healthy?

Who has time for that? Managing your own health can be that "one more thing" you can't squeeze into a day that's already filled up with doctor appointments, newly inherited household chores, and possibly your own job responsibilities.

Trudging up the Alzheimer's mountain can sap all your physical and emotional strength. But I am here to tell you that you must make it a priority to be healthy yourself in order to be an effective caregiver. This is not negotiable. How do you keep yourself healthy? You get help. You take classes. You talk to people who have been through this. You cannot do it alone, as I tried to do. The proof is in the numbers and illustrated by my own experience.

Consider this: people with Alzheimer's who are sixty-five and older survive, on average, four to eight years after their diagnosis. Some live with the disease as long as twenty years. When your caregiving burden means you give up a healthy lifestyle, you're stacking the odds against yourself, leaving you with the sickening possibility that your partner with Alzheimer's will outlive you. That's got to be one of the cruelest twists of this terrible disease.

Maybe you've read the "Twelve Steps for Caregivers" by Carol J. Farran and Eleanore Keane-Hagerty, who have studied and written about Alzheimer's and caregiving for years. It's based on the many twelve-step programs for people with addictions and has been around since 1989, when it was published in an Alzheimer's-related medical journal, and it still pops up on websites, blogs, and social media. Right there in black and white it says a caregiver should recognize this: "I need to take care of myself." It was good advice twenty-five years ago, and it's good advice today.

Think of the emergency instructions you get on an airplane—you have to put on your own oxygen mask before you can help others with theirs. No matter how much you love your partner, you can't take good care of him or her if you don't first take good care of yourself. I didn't realize how important that was until it was almost too late. I don't want that to happen to you.

What I wish I'd known

Chronic stress experienced by Alzheimer's caregivers may shorten their lives by as much as four to eight years.

When Elaine was well, and even after she first was diagnosed, I'd work out many weekday mornings with my friends. But as her mental decline continued, her body clock was affected, and that of course threw off my own sleep. If she was awake, I felt I should be awake too to make sure she wasn't wandering around or doing something unsafe. Sometimes, she'd ask and re-ask me questions but not any old questions. Instead, her queries packed an emotional punch. "Are we married?" "Do we have children?" "Do I have Alzheimer's?" "Is it bad?" "Why do I have it?" Just try getting back to sleep after that!

By the time we got up for the day, many times, she'd be confused and agitated . . . and I'd be exhausted and cranky. I simply couldn't leave her home alone in the morning to go to the health club. One missed workout led to another and another and . . . The theme from *Rocky*, the *William Tell* Overture, and "On Wisconsin" combined would not have been enough inspiration to push me out the door. Over the span of a year and a half, I put on twenty pounds.

Elaine, meanwhile, also put on weight, probably eight or ten pounds. Sometimes, she couldn't remember whether she'd eaten lunch. When in doubt, she'd make herself a peanut butter and jelly sandwich.

Carrying that extra weight—and I don't just mean the pounds—meant I couldn't even go up the stairs at home or my office without having to stop and catch my breath. Even when I was just walking, I often got short of breath. (My temper ran short, too . . . more on that in chapter 5.)

I already was a cancer survivor, having been diagnosed in 2006 with non-Hodgkin's lymphoma. I went through six cycles of chemotherapy over a six-month period with side effects that included low energy, nausea, and hair loss. Still, I remained confident that the treatment would work. And it did. So while I hated the idea of more clinics and exams for myself, I had to get some answers. The doctors quickly focused on a variety of heart issues.

Over a three-and-a-half-year span, from 2009 through late 2012, I underwent several procedures and also had a pacemaker installed. Still, I never felt quite right. I rang up more than $260,000 in medical bills as various doctors took their turns examining me, ordering tests and lab work, and even having me admitted. My wife was the one who was sick. Why was I the one in the hospital? My doctors blamed COPD (chronic obstructive pulmonary disease, a progressive lung disease), asthma, excess fluid in my upper chest, sleep apnea, and even a rare type of high blood pressure that affects arteries in the lungs and in the heart. Or maybe it was a combination of sheer exhaustion, acute anxiety, depression, and grieving.

No doubt about it, I was breaking down physically and emotionally. Would I ever learn to protect my own health? Yes, I wanted to take care of my wife, but I didn't want to be a dead hero. So, in December 2011, I finally contacted the Alzheimer's Association for help. Through the association, I met another Alzheimer's caregiver who became my mentor. He told me he'd had a heart attack, despite having no history of heart disease. That was all the wake-up call I needed. At long last, I was open to using the association's resources and suggestions.

What I wish I'd done

I should have started earlier to search out adult daycare so that I could reclaim part of the day for myself, including time for exercise.

Everyone is familiar with the concept of an adrenalin rush, a burst of energy that we associate with a startling, fight-or-flight event. It turns out other hormones also are released into the body in stressful situations. One of these is cortisol. It was useful to cavemen who had to outrun an attacking animal. But in our modern world, we rarely need that extra spurt of energy and actually find it works against our survival. When we live with constant stress, cortisol just keeps flooding into our bodies. Without physical activity or other stress-busters, the levels just stay high and wreak all sorts of havoc. According to the Mayo Clinic, stress is linked to heart disease, mental illnesses, digestive problems, sleep problems, weight gain, and—here's the ironic one for Alzheimer's caregivers—memory and concentration impairment. I've heard some health experts call chronic high stress a ticking time-bomb. At least now I know my enemy's name: cortisol.

Here's some more science. A team at Ohio State University and the federal National Institute of Aging spent nearly three decades investigating the links between psychological stress and a weakened immune system. The study, released in 2007, was much more than a survey. It included a comparison of blood samples of Alzheimer's caregivers to those of non-caregivers that revealed a difference at the genetic and molecular level. The scientists concluded that the chronic stress of Alzheimer's caregiving may shorten spouses' and children's lives by as much as four to eight years. Think about that: that's four to eight years you won't see your grandkids grow up.

The Mayo Clinic, Ohio State University, and the NIA aren't alone in looking at the possible links between Alzheimer's and caregiver health.

It's certainly a hot topic for anyone interested in health care reform and holding down expenditures. Back in 2010, economist Brent Fulton from the University of California, Berkeley, determined that Alzheimer's caregivers spend 8 percent more on health care than non-caregivers. In a more recent estimate, the Alzheimer's Association calculated that in 2015 the physical and emotional impact of dementia caregiving in the United States resulted in an estimated $10.2 billion—again, billion with a *b*—in health care costs.

As the research continues to reveal the unfortunate implications for the health of Alzheimer's caregivers, you continue to climb the Alzheimer's mountain.

To me, being an Alzheimer's caregiver is like being the fictional boxer Rocky Balboa in a pitched battle against a much stronger opponent. The disease can back you into a corner. You have to maintain your footing as you swing away. You're trying your damnedest to fight back while also struggling to control your own emotions. At the same time, you're absorbing some awful body blows like depression, anxiety, and grief. Each time there is another indication that your partner's mind is being affected, it's another blow.

Unlike Rocky, you'll never be able to defeat Alzheimer's, and if you're not careful, those blows, bit by bit, will defeat you in the trying. Work to understand the illness, and get the help and support you need to respond to it. That's the best path up the mountain.

[Marty] is on the phone with his office again. He does seem to miss the hustle and bustle of work more than enjoying everything here. I'm feeling he is not happy here and is needing more company than just me. I've convinced myself it is just the way it'll have to be. I'm happier here than at home, but I can tell he is missing his work place and probably his friends there.

— Elaine's Florida journal, dated March 28, 2012

—CHAPTER 4—
Isolation

*M*uch of the country probably thinks of Wisconsin *as a terribly cold place. Tune in to a Green Bay Packers game in December (or, hopefully, a home playoff game in January), and you'll see the Packers faithful bundled up in their snowmobile suits and parkas. Every time those eighty thousand fans exhale or shout their encouragement to their beloved team, you can see their breath. The stadium takes on an eerie energy as the breath vapors appear and then disappear into the cold air.*

The real frozen tundra, however, lies hundreds of miles north in places like Alaska and Canada's Northwest Territories—the inspiration for a rich culture.

One story that has emerged from Eskimo folklore tells of a practice (strange to us) for dealing with the sick elderly. During times of famine, food and other resources were stretched thin to take care of the young and healthy. That left little to spare for someone who wasn't contributing to the group—and the ill and elderly could be considered a burden to the rest of the community. So, the old person was taken to the edge of the sea, put on an ice floe, and pushed away from shore to drift away to die from exposure and starvation.

* * *

When your partner has Alzheimer's, you can feel as if you're the one living on an ice floe, isolated from anyone who cares about your well-being. In my case, feeling abandoned on a chunk of ice was a particularly precarious state to be in since I was gaining weight. Not only was I was floating away, I was also starting to sink!

If you have joint-replacement surgery or experience cancer (and I've done both), people respond to your immediate needs with understanding and empathy—and food—for the six weeks or six months that you're out of commission. Those acts of kindness are priceless. They fuel your physical healing and feed your spirit. If you're lucky, you reach the end of your rehab or chemo, and then you're able to do things for yourself again. You write thank-you notes, and everyone moves on.

I'd like to think that the weight gained during my early caregiving years was the result of friends and neighbors showering us with rich, home-delivered meals and decadent peach pies. But I'd be kidding myself. Alzheimer's is not a tuna-casserole disease. It's a years-long illness, traumatic for both the person with the disease and the caregiver, with no happy ending this side of heaven.

People don't usually think of offering rides or meals or help with the yard work to an Alzheimer's caregiver. Part of that is due to the fact that when you are a caregiver, you just don't interact with the outside world as much as you used to. Alzheimer's separates you from people you work with, play cards with, attend ballgames with, worship with—or, I should say, the people you *used* to do those things with before caregiving took over your life. They still love you, but they simply don't know how to respond.

Feeling so lonesome was something that I did not anticipate. It's like other negative aspects of caregiving— it silently creeps in on you. Caregivers, here is your warning: loneliness is coming your way. Its cousin, depression, might just show up on your doorstep, too.

Many people feel lonely occasionally. In one survey, 40 percent of people age sixty-five and older reported being lonely, at least sometimes. What do you suppose the figure is for Alzheimer's caregivers? I'm guessing 100 percent.

Loneliness itself is not a new topic of interest in the field of psychology. In 1978, researchers at UCLA first developed a twenty-item survey to determine a person's level of loneliness. It's still used today. Unlike the cognitive tests that help diagnose dementia, this test is self-administered. It asks, for example, how often you feel as if no one understands you and how often you feel isolated from other people. Does it make you feel any better if a quickie quiz tells you that you're lonely? Probably not.

Scientists and psychologists have done many studies on loneliness in recent years, and what they're learning is that loneliness is downright dangerous. In a University of Chicago study, lonelier people reported worse physical health, experienced more chronic diseases, and were more likely to develop coronary heart disease. Other research has linked loneliness to problems such as eating disorders, substance abuse, and even suicide. Yet another study, at Brigham Young University, concluded that loneliness damages your health almost as much as being obese or smoking fifteen cigarettes a day.

Loneliness is always a negative experience, according to Rose Beeson, a leading researcher on people who care for a spouse who has Alzheimer's. No kidding.

Heading off loneliness is a two-way street. You can't just put on a brave face day after day. You need to reach out to others and teach them about Alzheimer's. You can't be afraid of sounding like a whiner. To survive, you can't worry that you're being a burden.

And people need to reach out to you. They need to recognize how they can contribute to your well-being with those concrete offers of help.

In the early stages of Elaine's diagnosis, many people didn't know how to respond to our situation because she didn't look sick. They couldn't see what was causing the problem, that her brain was broken. She was struggling to make sense out of the world. I didn't look sick either, but I was suffering from a broken heart as I struggled to accept this awful new reality.

What I wish I'd known

The fact that family and friends can't fully understand what a caregiver is going through is not a good enough reason to avoid them.

I did try to keep things somewhat normal as the disease progressed. We had four or five couples with whom we often went out to dinner, and we did for two or three years after Elaine was diagnosed until she could no longer join in table talk about happenings around town or current events. It was so unfair to watch her put all that effort into social situations. Putting her in a position where she had to carry on a coherent conversation was as cruel as challenging someone on crutches to a tennis match.

For the next five or six years, the two of us did dine out a lot—for probably 90 percent of our meals—because even with my help Elaine couldn't so much as boil water (and I'm not much of a cook myself). She was always right across the table from me, yet those restaurant meals became increasingly sad experiences for me.

At home, there wasn't much to talk about, either. Earlier in the disease, Elaine had to resign from the boards of several organizations around town because she really couldn't participate in their activities. By the time she was in the middle stages of the disease (about five years after her diagnosis), she had lost all interest in reading, making photo albums, shopping, baking, housework, and so many other things she used to enjoy. She was anxious and bored.

Two of our four children live far from Milwaukee, several states away. Certainly, I kept all of them in the loop. But I didn't think it was helpful to over-dramatize the situation. You say, "Alzheimer's," and that's enough for your kids to understand the importance of spending time with Mom before she slips away completely. Each of them has handled the situation differently, and I can't say any of them has gotten it wrong.

The kids try their best to keep the connection with their mother alive. Naturally, it has become tougher as time passes. When you speak to someone face to face (whether they have dementia or not), eye contact and gestures communicate so much; of course, those things are missing over the phone. As Alzheimer's tightened its grip on Elaine's brain, she would repeat questions to the kids ("How are you?" "How is your family?"), sometimes five or six times. Ever hear someone say, "It's good just to hear your voice?" In this case, the voice was familiar, but Elaine's limited vocabulary was a painful reminder to our children that she was dying mentally. Naturally, the kids' calls became shorter and less frequent, and I can't blame them. Why call and have a continued painful experience?

My professional relationships were affected, too. Over the decades, I had worn out several sets of tires making the 160-mile round trip to the state capitol in Madison for various meetings and events. But now, I had no desire to work with members of the Wisconsin State Legislature—Republican or Democrat—on issues I should have cared about. I felt much better withdrawn than being involved. I was just too exhausted and too contented to stay home.

I didn't even budge during election season (which practically never ends in a battleground state like Wisconsin). Important people are always coming here for rallies and fund-raisers. Had I wanted to, I could have shared the stage with all sorts of Democratic Party dignitaries, including presidential and vice-presidential candidates. Government is in my blood, of course. My dad, Martin E. Schreiber, in addition to his thirty-two years as a Milwaukee alderman, also served one term in the Wisconsin Assembly. And I held political offices for sixteen years. For me to step away from the political arena was like a compulsive shopper staying home on Black Friday.

And remember all the skipped workouts that contributed to my health problems? Besides the exercise I missed out on, I was giving up my social interactions with that group of friends as well.

What I wish I'd done

From the beginning, I should have shared more information about Elaine and concerns about my ability to cope so that I could have begun to focus on surviving.

What I needed was someone to talk to about Alzheimer's. I needed someone to at least acknowledge the pain I was experiencing.

What I also needed was to *not* talk about Alzheimer's. I needed activities that focused my energy on my own interests and needs.

I needed to break the cycle of isolation that was eating me alive.

One other thing I needed: the ability to deal with mounting stress.

Marty is still a very good husband and I can't blame him for being a little short sometimes. It has to be a problem for him. It puts more responsibility than he can handle sometimes. But he knows I'm trying my best and tries hard to help me. I know it is no easier for him than for me.

— Elaine's notes during a visit to
Door County, Wisconsin, dated July 3, 2012

—CHAPTER 5—
Irrational Irritability

*E*ven though Alzheimer's was causing Elaine to behave *erratically, I decided we should go in 2011 to visit our daughter Kathy, who lives near Boston. When it came time to leave the hotel room, I discovered that, sometime while my back was turned, Elaine had unpacked all the luggage and returned items to the dresser drawers. She had done that at home before a trip, thinking she was being helpful. But now? When we needed to get to Logan International? Now the race was on to find and repack everything, and make it to the airport on time. With the clock ticking, our taxi raced to Logan; almost miraculously, we made it through security and to our gate just before they closed the door to the Jetway.*

We were the last people to board the plane and our two seats were the only ones left—at the back, naturally. I trudged down the aisle with Elaine following, relieved we'd made it but out of breath, each of us dragging a suitcase. Does it surprise you to learn that I couldn't get the bags to fit under the seat and that the overhead bins were closed?

I asked the flight attendant what to do with our bags, since the bins were full.

"You know," she replied, "we wouldn't have this trouble if you weren't the last people on the airplane."

Well, that lit my fuse! The anger welling up inside me came out as almost hatred. After all I had gone through to get us there on time, all this flight attendant could suggest was that we should have arrived earlier? Couldn't she see that I was desperately trying to catch my breath? "This has got to be," I declared, "the world's worst goddamn airline."

With that, the flight attendant rushed to the front of the plane to talk to her co-workers. As they looked back at me, I was sure they were discussing whether I was a threat to their safety and should be taken off the plane.

* * *

I like to think of myself as a pretty even-keeled guy. You have to have a thick skin to be in politics; it doesn't pay to get worked up about every little thing. My company's website brags about my charm and wit—hey, it's on the Internet so it must be true, right?

Charm and wit did not do me one iota of good on another trip, this time to Florida in November 2012. We planned to vacation there for the winter to escape the Wisconsin weather, so I took along cash to cover some meals and other expenses. A thousand dollars. It wasn't my best decision ever, but I put the cash in a jar on the dresser. Next day, it was gone. "Elaine, where is that money? Did you take that money?" For all I knew, she had flushed it down the toilet. A thousand dollars! Frantic and furious, I searched for those fifty-dollar and one-hundred-dollar bills everywhere. Buckets of cortisol must have been coursing through my body. Thankfully, four days later, I found the cash—stuffed into a sock in the dresser. It must have been Elaine's way of hiding it safely away, demonstrating once again that she could help. She had no idea of the consequences of her action.

What I wish I'd known

Unfamiliar settings such as hotels can be particularly upsetting to people with dementia because they have trouble re-orienting.

Honestly, I should have known better. Starting two or three years before this incident, I would find checks and cash stowed away in drawers and clothing all over our home in Milwaukee. When those things began happening, I took over all the management of our finances to keep things straight. Not only was it one more thing I had to tackle; it was also sad because Elaine had always handled all that so well—banking, credit cards, investing, charitable giving . . . the whole nine yards. As the disease took its toll, I was terrified that she might give away our life savings to telephone solicitors; thankfully, she didn't. One task she remained very good at was ordering packs of checks from our credit union—I found boxes with hundreds of newly printed checks. Looking on the bright side, that should cover us for a few years!

One more lost-item story. Once, Elaine put the car keys in the dishwasher. So, of course, the next time I couldn't find the keys, I assumed her helpful behavior was the explanation—she must have put them in her idea of a safe place—and I figured the next two hours of my life would be spent searching for those damn keys. (Yes, I did check the dishwasher, without success. People with Alzheimer's don't often put things away in the same place.) The blame game was already underway. This tale has a happy ending, though, with a twist. I learned it's best to not accuse your wife of hiding the car keys until you've checked your own coat pockets.

Something as big as nearly missing your flight or something as small as misplaced car keys gets magnified when you are an Alzheimer's caregiver. You are trying to do so much, and at the same time, you're dealing with sadness and grieving. Your instinct is to multitask your to-do list to death. If doing more than one thing at a time is something you can manage, all well and good. The risk comes in overloading yourself. When you can't give something your full attention, the result often is that you get less done, not more. That makes you tired, resentful, and crabby—a Grumpy Old Man, as it were.

I call this phenomenon "irrational irritability." You probably remember this emotion from those sleep-deprived days when your children were babies. Fortunately for parents, it's a lot easier to bounce back when you're in your twenties, thirties, or forties. And at least you know the sleepless nights aren't going to last forever.

An exhausted, stressed-out Alzheimer's caregiver who is sixty, seventy, or eighty years old, meanwhile, has a different threshold of anxiety. You get to the end of your rope quicker. Things that really shouldn't bother you, really do! This can lead to making poor decisions or saying hurtful things that you instantly regret. The last thing you want to do is drive people away, but it easily can happen. You don't want to know how many bouquets of flowers and boxes of candy I have given to friends, relatives, and even store clerks as peace offerings after losing my cool. Although I still believe that Boston flight attendant could have been far more helpful, maybe I should have sent flowers to her, too.

Sadly, some caregivers even lash out at their loved ones with dementia. Elder abuse has been a concern of mine going back to the early 1970s when as lieutenant governor I led a task force on overhauling Wisconsin's nursing home licensing and regulating system. Mistreatment of people who live in a care facility is a disgusting crime, and it goes on despite state and federal abuse-prevention laws—not to mention decency and common sense.

What I'm talking about here, though, is abuse and neglect by family members. Overall, 90 percent of those who abuse the elderly are family members, according to data compiled by the National Center on Elder Abuse. Researchers have also found that family members who abuse drugs and/or alcohol, who have a mental and/ or emotional illness, and who feel burdened by their caregiving responsibilities abuse at higher rates than those who are not in such situations.

When it comes to people with dementia, nearly half of their family caregivers (47.3 percent) were abusive, according to a study published in the Journal of the American Geriatrics Society. Verbal mistreatment is the most commonly reported type of abuse, by 60 percent of dementia caregivers. Next comes neglect, at 14 percent. And, unfortunately, 5 to 10 percent of caregivers are physically abusive toward a person with dementia.

Obviously, it's difficult to come up with accurate statistics because care recipients may be unable to talk about any abuse that is taking place and caregivers may not be truthful in answering questions about abusive behavior. But there is no question in my mind that family caregivers sometimes abuse someone with Alzheimer's or another form of dementia. We get irritable and sometimes behave irrationally. People who are hurting, hurt people.

And you are hurting. As your spouse's Alzheimer's progresses, you will face conversations that simply break your heart. You can't take it personally when your loved one can't remember names and events. When your curious, charming, four-year-old grandchild asks, "Why?" over and over, sure, it can get old. But when it's an adult yanking your chain (even though it's the disease talking), frustration is just a natural reaction. Ask any caregiver if he or she ever feels like screaming, and if the person is being honest, the answer is, "Yes . . . not only "feel like"; I *have* screamed!"

It's a very human thing to feel trapped and hopeless. Under stress and trying to adjust to—and accept—your new reality, it's very easy to pick at that scab. You flip your lid over something that would never bother you under normal circumstances. Of course you are angry. But be angry at the disease and not at your loved one.

Count to ten, walk away for a minute . . . do whatever it takes to get yourself calmed down.

To be the best—and most patient—caregiver possible, you need the right approach. It starts, as I explained in chapter 1, with recognizing that Alzheimer's is an enemy you cannot defeat. It continues, as I told you in chapter 3, with protecting your own health. It takes new strategies, such as perhaps putting your suitcases into the trunk of the car right away after you pack them.

It also takes letting go of being in control, as I'll describe in chapter 7. No one says you have to care alone.

What I wish I'd done

I should have paid more attention to reducing my stress so that I wouldn't become irrationally irritable, distracted, and forgetful.

I'll admit that, starting on this climb about ten years ago, I didn't know what Alzheimer's really was, how it would impact our lives, and how ill-equipped I was to take on the role of caregiver. Elaine and I were only in our mid-sixties when she began showing symptoms of cognitive impairment. We had expected to have many happy years to look forward to, but they were taken away from us. I felt cheated. I stubbornly held onto the Elaine that once was. I didn't always accept the obvious new normal, such as giving myself enough time to get the job done—and maybe re-done, if my wife unpacked my suitcase—that would head off a meltdown. I didn't enjoy losing control of my emotions. Every time I blew up, I swore it would be the last. If you were a victim of my irrational irritability, I apologize that you were the casualty of my hurt.

The resources and support of my local Alzheimer's Association chapter helped me finally pull it together. They nudged me into sharing my story in very public ways, such as this book, and that has helped me find a purpose in life. I hope my message is getting through to you, so you can be an effective caregiver and that you will learn, cope, and survive.

Coping with
Alzheimer's Disease

[I am] not enjoying my role any more as Marty's wife. Because of his having concerns about my Alzheimer's, he doesn't let me be me. Go for a walk if I want to, or to the store alone, etc., etc. I used to appreciate him—what I thought was concern—but he holds me captive much too much. I am going to try to have a second opinion because I really don't think I have any problem. I know how to drive or walk anyplace I want to enjoy but he doesn't believe me and I hate the control he has placed on me. I don't even think I have Alzheimer's per se.

— Elaine's journal, 2009

—CHAPTER 6—
Reaching for a Lifeline

A woman had a parrot. All day long, for hours, for years, the parrot would repeat, "Polly wants a party. Polly wants a party." The woman was expecting some very important company and became very concerned about the image she would project if her parrot would squawk, "Polly wants a party. Polly wants a party," while she entertained her distinguished guests.

At her wit's end, the woman went to her priest to ask for advice. The good father could hardly believe the coincidence—he himself had two parrots, Peter Parrot and Paul Parrot. What was so very special about these birds, he explained, was that for many years his parrots would fervently pray. Pray from morning to night, every waking hour.

The priest suggested that the woman bring Polly to the church to meet Peter and Paul. He was sure his pious parrots would provide the powerful, positive influence that Polly so obviously needed.

With great hope, the woman hurried home and retrieved Polly. Predictably, as soon as the parrot was put into the cage with the priest's birds, she loudly screeched, "Polly wants a party. Polly wants a party."

With that, Peter Parrot looked at Paul Parrot and said, "Our prayers have finally been answered!"

* * *

Finding the right way to provide for Elaine's changing needs over the course of climbing this Alzheimer's mountain has required persistence and determination, the likes of which I did not know I could muster.

Long before I recognized that I needed help as a caregiver, Elaine and I were working together to find the best ways to maintain her quality of life. As I mentioned earlier, when she first was diagnosed in 2007, she devoted her energy to reading all she could about Alzheimer's. We stayed busy with walks and time with friends. That was not enough.

Through her own research, Elaine affirmed how important it was to exercise. That led to her identifying a nearby community center that had an indoor pool. Elaine thought this would be an ideal way to stay in good physical shape and do something positive for herself. You didn't even have to sign up for a membership—just pay as you go—so there was no pressure. Elaine, who had been a lifelong swimmer, soon was going there three mornings a week and making friends. The center also offered massage therapy, including Reiki. Elaine had read that massage helped both the body and the mind relax, so she added that to her schedule once a week. She even drove herself there; after all, it was barely three minutes from home.

For several months, it really was perfect. Unfortunately, her symptoms were gradually getting worse.

That's how Alzheimer's is. You think you have this thing figured out, and then you don't.

A symptom that began to take hold of Elaine was excessive shopping. To support its many programs, the community center operated a sort of thrift store and gift shop. Costume jewelry, shirts, skirts, blouses, sweaters, glassware, books, movies, candle holders, even eight-track tapes . . . they all began finding their way into our home. She never came home empty-handed! It took me awhile to understand why all this buying was so important to her. I concluded that she thought she had to do her part to help this community center succeed. Since then, I learned that hoarding is one of the behaviors people with dementia might exhibit; experts say it can stem from the person's fear that they may need the items someday.

Around this time, the bigger problem for Elaine was that driving was increasingly more difficult. Even though the pool was just a mile and a half down the street, she was getting lost. This upset her and was obviously unsafe for her as well as anyone else on the road. Fortunately, she was able to continue going to the center for a while, thanks to a neighbor who provided her rides; sometimes, I drove her.

As I waited for her at the center, I learned that it also offered adult day services and a specialized program for people with dementia. Elaine might not need five-days-a-week services, but maybe a couple of days would benefit us both. Staff members saw that I was having trouble breathing and told me of their concern. The social worker could tell that my spirit was suffering, too. It was obvious to them that I needed some more "me" time, more than the hour I got during Elaine's swim or massage.

What the outside world didn't see was that I was beginning to lean more and more on what I call the "caregivers' poison"—alcohol—as a way to cope with my sad situation. I would reach five in the afternoon and consider myself successful for having made it through another day. I wasn't brimming with pride; I was just relieved and thinking that maybe my worries were behind me for a few hours. Time to relax with a drink or two.

It was, in a way, comforting. Not only did the alcohol numb my mind; it also helped me escape the reality. I felt calmer, more at ease. My evenings were not marked by the irrational irritability, which caused me so much trouble at times during the day. Drinking also enabled me to fall asleep quite easily. Although once the alcohol wore off a bit during nighttime, it was back to awake awareness and restless nights of interrupted sleep.

The reality is, of course, that all the armies marching and all the navies sailing cannot at this time stop Alzheimer's. So also, drinking all the beer brewed and all the whiskey aged cannot change the course of this disease. Alcohol use can be the caregivers' curse. It has to be recognized and dealt with. Otherwise, there is one more monster—quite an ugly one at that—to make life more difficult for both the caregiver and the person with dementia.

I was fortunate in that I was a "short hitter." Plus, our daughter Kristine was tuned in to the situation and talked with me about it. She also provided me an article on the benefits of moderate drinking; be assured that it was not given to me because I was drinking too little. My doctor became concerned as well and told me I was over self-medicating, to put it politely. (I still work to limit my drinks to two a day. Most times I succeed.)

With all this playing in the background, I wanted Elaine to at least try a day program, so I could get some respite.

This could have been our turning point. But Elaine would have no part of it.

Sadly, we left that community center just a few months later when swimming no longer was a suitable activity for Elaine and left behind whatever help it could have offered. We were on our own again.

I thought the answer to our situation might be to bring help into our home. I contacted a home care agency. That was tricky because Elaine was adamantly opposed to any professional caregivers invading her turf. Women can be pretty protective of their kitchens, and people with Alzheimer's can have an even more difficult time with someone else being in their home. They can be very distrustful of strangers and even of friends and family. They may even accuse people of stealing, which partially explains why someone with dementia tends to move (hide) valuables.

The first couple of in-home helpers suggested by the agency were younger women. That really made Elaine uncomfortable. I tried someone more her age, but that was no better. Not to be so easily defeated, I kept trying. I attempted to explain to Elaine that the home care wasn't for her, saying it was for me, but she told me, "That's your problem." So next I tried lying (more on that in chapter 8). I made up a story that this lady (actually the caregiver) was new in town. She wanted someone to walk her around the neighborhood and show her where different businesses, parks, and churches were and to help her find her way around a new grocery store. I thought that was pretty clever. Whether or not Elaine saw through my story, it didn't succeed. She declared that this new-lady-in-town's difficulties were not her responsibility. This defiant attitude was in sharp contrast to Elaine's usually gracious personality.

All told, the community center experience and my attempts to have care provided for Elaine in our home consumed more than a year after her diagnosis. Obviously, Elaine's symptoms were getting worse. I still had not accessed caregiver support of any kind; my focus was on what would benefit Elaine. I started looking for another option.

What I wish I'd known

The Alzheimer's Association has information on local programs and care centers. On alz.org, find the search field at the top of the home page, and type in "community resources."

I'd heard that a care facility in town offered an adult daycare program for people in the early stages of memory loss, and I thought it was worth checking out. Elaine already was familiar with this facility because her mother had spent the final years of her life there. Fortunately, Elaine was agreeable to going one day a week to what we called "continuing education." By the grace of God, she did not associate this program with dementia care.

Elaine was "going to classes," and indeed dutifully took a college-rule notebook with her and made use of it every week. The staff and volunteers helped small groups of participants play games and do memory exercises. Elaine became almost obsessed with journaling every part of the experience. One time, the group went on a field trip to a candy factory in a town about an hour away. Her notebook covered the bus ride in remarkable detail, with highlights of many street corners and nearly exact turn-by-turn directions.

Elaine also kept a journal when we were in Florida over the winter of 2011-2012. By then she got her days mixed up easily. I did my best to help her keep things straight, but I didn't always have time for her questions because I was busy on my laptop or phone tending to business matters back home. So, I bought her a special digital clock that clearly displayed the date and day of the week, as well as the time. She also referred to the newspaper each day to help her keep track of the calendar. A byproduct of that routine was that she was well aware of the upcoming presidential election—she mentioned it over and over in her vacation journal, the cover of which featured a whimsical scene of several dogs seated on porch chairs overlooking the beach.

But before we had traveled to Florida in 2011, something quite significant had happened that fall.

Although I was convinced that we already had gone to enough doctors—there had been at least four since 2005—Elaine wanted to be seen by a woman doctor. Completely on her own, without my knowledge, she made a call to the Alzheimer's Association's 24/7 Helpline (1-800-272-3900) in search of a suggestion. Meanwhile, in another part of the association's Southeastern Wisconsin offices, work was well underway to plan the annual "Walk to End Alzheimer's." At that time, one of the walk's organizers told the staff that she desperately needed a person with early-stage dementia to speak at the fundraiser because the original speaker had just cancelled. With Elaine's permission, the helpline counselor shared her first name with the walk organizer, who then contacted Elaine. In that conversation, Elaine disclosed that she was Elaine Schreiber, the former First Lady of Wisconsin. When asked to participate, Elaine told her, "I will be a public face of this disease," and within a week, she was appearing on local TV to promote the walk.

On the cool, sunshiny day of the walk, Elaine wore an official purple T-shirt, a red baseball cap, and the biggest, friendliest smile you can imagine. She proudly stood onstage to show the world that a person with early-stage Alzheimer's looks like anybody else. When she took the microphone, she thanked the participants for coming and urged them to get involved with the association. Her remarks were brief and well-delivered; as you might expect, she had written them out in advance. A college campus, a crowd of thousands, let's-get-fired-up music over the loudspeaker—the event had all the trappings of a political rally, only this time it was Elaine who was the center of attention.

By reaching out, not only had Elaine received the referral she sought, but also the association came to know her. An invaluable relationship was established. Lines of communication were opened that began to change our lives. It is no exaggeration to describe Elaine's initial phone call to the helpline as monumental and transformative.

A year later in October 2012, we were back at the Walk to End Alzheimer's with my firm's name printed on the back of the T-shirts as a sponsor.

Before we returned to Florida in November 2012, our dear friends Don and Karen, who lived in the vacation condo next door to ours, had researched adult-care programs in the area. They even visited four or five places before we arrived; they helped me choose a program that would meet Elaine's needs. If you can believe our good fortune, it was located only about a mile away, and was operated by a Lutheran church.

What I wish I'd done

I should have worked to find a healthy outlet for my own sadness and fearfulness, so that anticipatory grief wouldn't limit my day-to-day functioning.

By the time we came back to Wisconsin in April 2013, Elaine was so accustomed to attending "classes" that she was ready for a program that met every weekday. Together, we toured a facility near downtown Milwaukee and met with several staff members. To a person, they were positive, smiling, and courteous. It's a good thing Elaine was so willing to go there. Even after a winter in the warm Florida sun, I was more and more in need of respite time.

Five mornings a week, she'd fuss with her hair and makeup before we headed to breakfast. She was armed with her spiral notebook, of course, when I took her to "class" for the day, usually around 9:00 a.m. I would pick her up again at 3:00 or 3:30 in the afternoon.

I wish I could say that the weekday program put an end to my daily stress. It did buy me a few hours to do some household chores, maybe get in some exercise or tackle some of my company's work that had been pushed off to the side for so long. The problem was the black cloud of Alzheimer's that followed me everywhere. My mind remained busy with thoughts of what the disease was doing to Elaine and what surely was coming. There was a growing and unavoidable sense of foreboding.

I wish my Alzheimer's would dissipate. I'd like to be the smart wife and mother I used to be. Now, I have to waste so much time just trying to figure out what I should be doing—without seeming as smart as I used to be. I need to rely on Marty for everything. And I'm very lucky he continues to keep me. Life gets more difficult every day.

— A note by Elaine, date unknown

—CHAPTER 7—
Being a Real Man

After I lost the race for governor in 1978, we moved to a hobby farm in central Wisconsin. I had always loved horses as a child. Man, how I lived for the one-hour-a year horseback ride my parents would treat me to at the Kettle Moraine State Forest, an hour from Milwaukee. So, this move was my chance to buy a horse. Her name was Brianna, but for the purpose of this story—to make it more exciting—I will use the name Thunderbolt Killer.

I got a great bargain when I bought this mare since she wasn't fully broken to the saddle. I hired a trainer to help me every Saturday morning. Between sessions, I'd work on the skills we had learned before something new was introduced. One Saturday, the trainer took a rope and tied one end to the halter on her head and the other to the horse's tail—she was connected to herself in a sort of turned position. Thunderbolt Killer just stood there. "This is one smart horse," the trainer said. "Most horses would buck and jump, but you've got one that's first trying to *figure out how it got into this predicament and how to get out of it."*

* * *

With Alzheimer's caregiving, there's no point in bucking and jumping whenever you find yourself in a difficult situation. That only creates more havoc. You need to be smart. How did I get into this predicament, and how am I going to untangle myself safely? The answer is it didn't happen overnight, and you're going to need a lot of help.

What follows applies also to wives taking care of their husbands, but the shift in roles is often more challenging for men who become caregivers. This is because men have to learn so many new skills and travel through unfamiliar emotional territory as they climb the Alzheimer's mountain. So I will speak very bluntly to you husbands. You and your wife have always been a team, building each other's careers and sharing in the work of raising a family. Now, the balance will shift little by little until you'll be taking care of her a lot more than she takes care of you. You'll do all the driving. You'll go to all her doctors' appointments and manage her medications. You'll take over the housework, shopping, and cooking. You'll choose her clothing and help her get dressed. You'll help her safely take a shower and, eventually, even help her use the toilet.

You'll do all that—and much more—with a broken heart. I know that your natural instinct is to try carrying this weight alone. Being a real man means being brave, suffering in silence, and standing on your own two feet. Right? You're not supposed to depend on others, are you? There's a lot of truth in the old stereotype that male drivers don't like to stop and ask for directions. But to be a good caregiver, asking for help is exactly what you have to do. That's how you show how strong you are.

Before Alzheimer's, I'd spent a lifetime in politics and business delegating responsibility to my staff and employees. Somehow, dealing with this disease was different. For many months, I wasn't very public about Elaine's diagnosis and how I was being impacted. I guess I didn't want to unload on people beyond the circle of our closest friends. Stubborn, stupid Marty!

There's no shame in your spouse having Alzheimer's, and there's no shame in your asking for help. The sooner I had spent time in a support group, the sooner I'd have known that. When I finally did reach out to the Alzheimer's Association, about four years into my climb up this caregiving mountain, I began meeting with a counselor at my local chapter's office. She put me in contact with other caregivers, who I found easy to talk to one on one. Collectively, they helped me understand that you can't go it alone.

Did you catch that? It took me FOUR YEARS to begin working with the Alzheimer's Association to get the help I needed. During those four years, I had health problems that possibly could have been avoided. I don't want you to wait anywhere near that long to take advantage of the association's support.

I know I am repeating myself, but I feel I have to do that because my message is so important: get help. Take out your phone right now, and put the Alzheimer's Association Helpline number (1-800-272-3900) into your contacts list. Remember: it's a free, 24/7 resource that offers information about the disease, treatment options, caregiver skills, and much more.

What I wish I'd known

Asking others to help does not mean you're not strong enough or not trying hard enough.

When it comes to having someone to turn to, let's face it, most men don't have as many close friends as women do. But whether man or woman, if you are the primary caregiver, take a minute right now, and name three people outside your family whom you confide in.

This isn't like Facebook where you might have hundreds of "friends." I'm talking about the true-blue friends who will listen long enough to know what it's really like to be married to someone who has Alzheimer's. Even if your list is three people—or especially if you can't come up with that many—you need to reach out to the Alzheimer's Association. They'll help you.

One thing that makes it hard to ask friends for help is that Alzheimer's makes most people uncomfortable. Few people understand what it's about, other than to know it's not good. In fairness to my friends, they, too, are grieving the loss of the First Elaine. For the longest time, I was satisfied just to have a friend ask, "What can I do?" The offer itself was comforting. You might even say it's like having a million dollars in the bank. But that million-dollar account doesn't mean anything if you don't spend fifty bucks now and then.

It seems obvious, but every hour not spent on errands or chores is time you have for other things—whether it's something your wife needs or taking better care of yourself. What's on your to-do list? Could someone else buy a few groceries this week? Drop off dry-cleaning? Return library books? Walk the dog? Run your car through the car wash? Or bring you a tuna casserole?

With a better comprehension of how Alzheimer's was affecting Elaine, I would have known what kind of help to ask for. For example, when Elaine was in the early stages of the disease, I could have requested that a friend take her for a walk or out for coffee. She usually did better in one-on-one situations where little was expected of her. I enjoyed those times, and I bet her friends would have, too.

What I wish I'd done

I should have enlisted a couple of friends to be my team captains who could do the asking and scheduling for me.

And, I could have had some respite time when our children visited from out of town. They certainly were willing to help. But I still considered their visits to be occasions to entertain them and take care of them as Elaine and I had done for the previous twenty years. What I really needed, however, was to rest. It wasn't until I was so physically worn out that I finally allowed myself the luxury to sleep in or grab a nap while they were here to help with Elaine. I shouldn't have pretended for so long that I was doing fine.

There are lots of ways to recruit and organize your helpers. You can set up a personalized schedule online, using the Care Team Calendar on the Alzheimer's

Association website (find it on the Caregiver Center page). On the calendar, you list what kind of help you need and when, and friends can sign up to volunteer. You can find websites with similar tools on the Internet, including Lotsa Helping Hands, CareCalendar and CaringBridge.

Be sure you have current e-mail addresses and phone numbers for people who might be able to help. Send out a group message ("Dear friends, please excuse my manners in not asking you face to face, but I am having a difficult time managing all the things I need to do . . . "). If technology isn't your thing, see if a friend will organize a phone tree or mail out a letter to some of your friends. As the word gets around, I know you will get offers of help.

For the first four years—four long years—as I hiked the Alzheimer's trail, I stuck to my crazy notion that I didn't need anyone's map or suggestions. I believed that as long as I loved Elaine (and I'd had a half-century of practice at that already), I could handle the rest. Thank heaven I finally realized how wrong I had been. Look at what my attitude cost me—aggravation, good health, lost moments of joy with Elaine, and a friend or two along the way. Caregiver burnout and loneliness feed on each other. Admit you need help. Then get it.

Everyone but [Marty] tells me how well I'm doing and [I] always hear I should continue doing everything I have been—as most of my friends tell me I am doing well and if they didn't know I had Alzheimer's wouldn't know. I too feel that I am as normal as most people in their seventies.

— Elaine's notes during a visit to
Door County, Wisconsin, dated July 3, 2012

—CHAPTER 8—

Therapeutic Fibbing:
Entering Her Reality

A man is out driving one afternoon and comes across an injured pedestrian in the roadway. He knows that medical care is needed immediately, so he calls 9-1-1 and frantically tells the operator, "You've got to send help right away to Pistachio Street."

The operator says, "How do you spell Pistachio?" The man says, "I don't know! What I do know is he needs the EMTs!!"

The operator says, "I'm sorry, I can't dispatch the ambulance without inputting in the correct street name on my computer."

"OK," says the man. "I'll call you back in five minutes."

"Five minutes! Why five minutes?" asks the operator.

The man replies, "I'm going to drag the guy a block over to Elm Street."

* * *

The stark reality is if your partner ever did know how to spell *pistachio*, he or she won't for long.

When cognitive problems first start to show, you'll find yourself trying to fill in the gaps, providing a detail your partner is trying to recall, or prompting with a word he or she can't come up with on his or her own. "Old age," you tell yourself.

Then, you find out it's Alzheimer's.

The greater stark reality is that conversations are going to get only more difficult. You might be tempted to jump in more than ever before to fill in the blanks. It takes a lot of patience to hold yourself back and give your partner a chance to make the point, even if he or she is wrong. Know this: you cannot argue with Alzheimer's and expect to win.

Trying to set your spouse straight when he or she gets a detail wrong in some old family story is an exhausting exercise. It can turn into a disagreement that's completely unnecessary. Is it really important that you two went to the seafood place, not the steakhouse, to celebrate your partner's fiftieth birthday?

Your partner may not remember actually having a fiftieth birthday. One time, Elaine asked, "How old am I?" Rather than chiding her for not knowing, or even giving her a straight answer, I asked, "How old do you want to be?" And we had a good laugh.

Elaine at age six.

LEFT: Classmates selected Elaine as Miss Basketball, an honor similar to Homecoming Queen, when we were seniors in 1957. CENTER: Elaine hand-painted my campaign posters in 1954. I'm so glad she kept one in a scrapbook all these years. RIGHT: Our high school was so strict that it did not allow dances. Roller-skating parties, like this one in 1956, were the next-best thing. BOTTOM: College Spring Break, 1958.

My beautiful bride made her own dress. We were married on June 3, 1961, in Milwaukee.

LEFT: Pausing with baby Kathy in the doorway of our first house, on Monroe Street, in 1962. RIGHT: On the campaign trail for lieutenant governor in 1966 with our son Marty and daughter Kathy. BOTTOM: Elaine, Patrick Lucey, and I got to meet Bobby Kennedy at a fundraiser in 1966.

Our daughter Kristine did the honors pinning on my boutonniere prior to my swearing-in as lieutenant governor in 1971. At right are Jean Lucey and Governor Patrick Lucey. Jean also struggled with Alzheimer's disease; she died in 2011.

LEFT: At my office in the Capitol with our kids, Kathy, Kristine, Marty, and little Matt, in 1978. RIGHT: A light moment with Matt during the 1978 election campaign. BOTTOM: Elaine took a turn on the White House dance floor with President Carter in 1978.

TOP: Sailing – moments of joy – 1985. BOTTOM: Reading a bedtime story to grandkids Maurie, Jesse, and Virginia in 1999.

LEFT: "They're with us" reads Elaine's T-shirt, a gag gift when we got all four kids together in 2010. *From left to right*, Matt, Kathy, Kristine, and Marty.

RIGHT: Posing with Tom Hlavacek of the Alzheimer's Association before Elaine's speech at the Walk to End Alzheimer's in 2011.

Elaine and I shared this moment of joy in October 2015 at her memory care assisted living facility.

For your own sanity, get rid of the idea that you are always right. Lose the attitude! Do you want to be right, or do you want to be happy? You are now living in two realities: your partner's and yours. Spending time in that Alzheimer's reality is an important way to demonstrate your love.

Neuroscientists at UCLA—coincidentally, the same university that developed the loneliness scale I mentioned a few chapters ago—studied images of the brain and concluded that loving relationships actually alter the brain in positive ways. Essayist Diane Ackerman calls it the brain on love. "When your brain knows you're with someone you can trust," she writes, "it needn't waste precious resources coping with stressors or menace." Of course, that's not to say that you can love away someone's dementia. We all wish it were that simple.

When you try to reason with someone who has Alzheimer's, it only intensifies the trouble (and activates your stress hormones). You've got to remind yourself that while your partner looks the same on the outside, things are very different on the inside. Dementia is transforming the world into a reality unfamiliar to you. Especially in the late stages of Alzheimer's, a person with dementia is happier in his or her own world. Your job is to keep your partner's mind at ease, so he or she feels safe and loved. One Alzheimer's caregiver calls it "compassionate communication."

There's just no good reason to correct Elaine when she thinks I've been in Madison on business all day when in fact I've been in Milwaukee the whole time. The truth is out there, as they say, but it simply isn't important. I join along with her and enjoy the conversation. I might retell a short story about something special that happened when we lived in Madison or just agree with her. "Yes, honey, I was in Madison, and the traffic coming back was a real mess."

This concept is "therapeutic fibbing." I have to admit, that sounds better than "providing false testimony," as my dusty old law school textbooks would call it. And it's a lot more palatable than "lying," which is what people think politicians do most of the time. Imagine if I'd known this was an option fifty-five years ago when we were first married or in my campaigns for governor and mayor!

Getting serious again, I've discovered that, when you can tell that little white lie, it's a means to a more peaceful relationship with someone who has Alzheimer's. I call it therapeutic, because it's a tonic that tamps down some of the pain with which you are living.

What I wish I'd known

You're a healthier, happier, and more helpful caregiver if you are less confrontational.

Fibbing is a useful tactic when a person with dementia asks about family members and friends. A woman in her natural role as a nurturer or a man in his customary role as a provider will always be concerned about the people he or she loves. How is my dad? Is my brother all right? A parent will wonder and worry about his or her children. As the ability to process and remember information diminishes, your job is to deflect your partner's fears and concerns.

"Are our kids doing OK?" you'll be asked—probably over and over.

"Yes, everyone's fine," you'll respond.

I once made the terrible mistake of answering one of Elaine's questions about her parents by telling her the truth, that they were dead. She looked as sad as the day many years earlier when she learned they had died.

"Dead?" she repeated, concerned and puzzled. "Did we take good care of them? Did I go to their funerals?"

She was distraught to think that maybe she hadn't honored them properly. What good did it do to give her a real-world answer when she lives in her own altered world? Until I saw the sorrow in her eyes, I didn't know that the truth wasn't always relevant. I vowed I wouldn't put her through that kind of pain again. Sometime later, we heard a piece of music that made her think of her folks; she remarked that they *would* enjoy it (present tense). Not that they *would have* enjoyed it (past tense).

This time, I responded in the way I now knew was better for her. "They sure would," I told her.

More recently, with Alzheimer's continuing to squeeze the memory out of Elaine's brain, she told me something odd yet sweet. It was a statement I didn't dare dispute. In fact, I took it as a great compliment. She said, "You look just like my husband."

Another very helpful approach is "redirecting." The idea is to change the focus of the person with dementia, thereby preventing a conversation from turning into an argument. For instance, when Elaine asks me for a glass of wine at 9:00 a.m., there's no point in giving her the dozen reasons why that's not happening. Instead, I shift the discussion to other things related to wine. For instance, I talk about how pretty wine looks in its glass or ask who else she would like to drink wine with. After a few minutes of that, she's moved on. Use your partner's framework (here, the wine) and redirect to another subject (in this case, wine glasses and friends).

What I wish I'd done

I should have used my wife's frame of reference instead of challenging it.

Tense situations also can come up because a person with Alzheimer's increasingly has trouble relating to logical boundaries. Dementia can cause someone to pick things up unnecessarily and move them. (You do remember the panic that resulted from the suitcase-unpacking incident and the misplaced-cash fiasco.) Or it could be that your partner picks up something that doesn't belong to him or her. Maybe he wants to put on someone else's sweater instead of his own, or at dinner, she reaches for the wrong glass. You can waste time and energy to try to correct your partner, or you can let it go. Ask yourself, does it matter? Is anyone at risk of injury? If others are with you, make sure they understand what is going on, explain the best response in such situations, and advise them to accept this as normal for Alzheimer's. Help them so you all can let it go!

Better yet, thank your partner for "finding" the sweater or glass you'd been "looking for." Not only have you avoided a confrontation, but you also have given that person an opportunity to feel proud of himself or herself. To feel useful. To hear in your voice and see in your facial expression that you're grateful for the help.

Therapeutic fibbing and redirecting are two of the best ways I've found to keep stress from consuming me. They've also given me the opportunity to turn a potential "I'm right, you're wrong" conversation into a moment of joy. It's all part of knowing how Alzheimer's plays out. It's a way to cope.

Life is better than ever. Even my knee is cooperating and Marty, too. He's finally relaxing more. We took our morning walk and saw at least ten little lizards along the way. Nature has a way of making you appreciate life—including our wonderful human time together.

— Elaine's Florida journal, dated April 5, 2012

CHAPTER 9

Living in the Now

There is a story about a wise Indian chief who was blind. They say he had the wisdom of Solomon. One day, two young braves came up with a plan to trick the chief and show that he was not so wise or intelligent.

They decided to go before the chief with one of them holding a sparrow in his hand and ask the chief if the sparrow was dead or alive. If the chief were to say the sparrow was dead, the brave would open his hand and let the bird fly away. If the chief said the sparrow was alive, the brave would crush the bird in his hand; the sparrow would be dead. Either way, the chief would be wrong.

With that plan, the braves went before the chief with one of them holding the sparrow.

"Chief," he said, "I have a sparrow in my hand. Is it dead or alive?"

The chief responded, "The sparrow is as you choose it to be, as you wish it to be."

* * *

The choices you make dictate how successful you may be in your caregiving. Many times, you can influence the outcome by controlling the moment, by living in the moment of a person with dementia.

Experts say that exercise is one way to hold off the Alzheimer's monster banging its way out of your closet. It makes sense—do something that raises your heart rate, and more blood flows to your brain. In fact, Elaine's doctor says walking is the best exercise for the brain of both a person with Alzheimer's and his or her caregiver.

With that advice in mind, we set out one day on the paved bicycle path behind our condo for a walk. Elaine didn't have an agenda. There was no pressure to achieve a goal during what ought to be a perfectly enjoyable event on its own and no awareness of whether we'd been on that bike path for twenty-one or twenty-three or twenty-nine and a half minutes. However, she was well aware of how tall the trees were, how pretty the flowers were, that there was a butterfly, and that leaves were blowing in the breeze. Her interest was to take in nature's wonders and appreciate them Zen-like and in the moment.

My goal was to walk from A to B in thirty minutes, to get it done, and go on with my day.

Checking my watch, mentally moving on to whatever was next on my to-do list when we got home— that was my misguided focus. How foolish of me! I had missed a moment of joy. *We* had missed out. The sooner you choose to acknowledge the disease, the sooner you begin to identify and enjoy those moments. It is your choice to enjoy the process—of walking or whatever—without focusing on the end result. I definitely could have made better decisions. I'm telling you, don't wait until it's too late.

So, if it's a beautiful day for a walk, do that. But when the walk is actually happening, it is your choice either to let an arbitrary fitness standard rule the day or, instead, to capture that moment of joy. I hope you choose to enjoy the moment and snap the mental picture that you can always hold.

Remember the cognitive tests that Elaine was given? She started out with a score of twenty-eight out of thirty points on one assessment. But as the score goes down, caregiving responsibilities increase and there is more that demands an attentive response. It's like watching the temperature drop—the colder it gets, the more layers of clothing you need. When you are prepared, moments of joy happen more easily. When you are not prepared, brace yourself for moments of frustration.

While no two people with Alzheimer's experience the disease in exactly the same way, it is in the late stages that a person undergoes the greatest changes in physical abilities. Bicycling was a hobby that Elaine and I had enjoyed over the years, and of course that bike path behind our condo is so conveniently located. They say you never forget how to ride a bike, right? Well, they're wrong. Elaine got to the point where she could no longer ride a bike.

So, we went to a bicycle shop that sold three-wheel models, designed for adults with balance difficulties. Elaine was successful sitting on the bike, but because her Alzheimer's was so far advanced, she couldn't relate to the handlebars. She could not comprehend that if you wanted to go straight you held the handlebars steady in front of you. "This is stupid," she announced, getting off the bike. I had no idea how dramatically she could decline. By the time I thought of the three-wheeler, her tests were scoring in the low teens. The disease was just progressing too quickly.

What I wish I'd known

Alzheimer's is a disease of inactivity of both mind and body. As it progresses, the person with the disease becomes slower and less capable. You can try familiar activities, but you need to accept when the brain can no longer process the information.

Trying to get Elaine to ride that bike when I did was my living in the past. It was as illogical as expecting her to be able to handle trips to Boston and Florida. I had lived such an active life with my First Elaine. With my Second Elaine, that is no more. Unfortunately, it took me too long a time to realize that I must choose to let go, to accept that hard truth. We still can experience happiness, but like Dorothy in *The Wizard of Oz*, we must find it right in our own backyard.

One of the most painful losses for couples affected by Alzheimer's is not being able to really talk about the kids and grandkids. Milestones such as graduations, weddings, and births come and go. Sadly, a person with Alzheimer's is unable to be truly involved. For them, those family members might as well be strangers off the street.

Knowing that, I still do tell Elaine about our children and grandchildren. It's still worth doing. She might not be able to relate to the characters in my stories all the time, but she can sense that these are people I love and am proud of. She can feel the joy I am expressing. It's not the details of the stories that are important; it's the mood that is created by telling them.

That's my way of slaying the dragon—choosing to see my wife as the person she is now. Helping her enjoy the person she is now. Helping her sense that I am happy to be with her now. I've finally learned to slow down and appreciate the moments of joy, however fleeting they might be. Thankfully, most of the time she still knows me and always remarks about how good-looking and intelligent I am. Who wouldn't want to hear that?

I never want to pass up the opportunity to tell Elaine how pretty she is, how wonderful she is, what a good person she is. She likes that. Sometimes when I do that, she calls me a BSer again, but we both laugh and enjoy the moment. Her smile tells me she is in a good place.

The person my wife is now finds happiness in lots of things. We listen to music and sing. We play catch. We play board games without rules. We color—we were way ahead of that coloring-books-for-adults fad! And we make simple art projects. (An Alzheimer's Association program called Memories in the Making helps persons with the disease express themselves through art. The watercolor paintings they create are remarkable and so good they can sell at auction for several hundred dollars.)

What I wish I'd done

By wishing for the past, I had deprived my wife of happiness in the moment. Even though it broke my heart, I should have let go of my First Elaine sooner, so I could love my Second Elaine where she is now.

I know Elaine benefits from the comfort and security that comes from just being with me and other people who love her, including the people she gave her life to. Everyone deserves that bit of dignity, regardless of his or her mental condition. I still need her, and she somehow knows that. She's sensitive and aware of her surroundings. After fifty-five years of marriage, she's closely tuned into my attitude, frustration, and impatience; she just seems to know precisely what emotional state I am in.

We spend a lot of time just looking out the window. It's an experience much like that walk on the bike path. "Look at that tree. It's so big!" "The sky is so blue." "Those are pretty flowers." And then we start over with our little survey of nature until she finally loses interest. You have to grasp each of those statements and appreciate them individually, not dread the tedium of it. What she had for dinner isn't on her mind right now—it's that the tree is big, the sky is blue, the flowers are pretty.

Go to your kitchen or your workbench, get a funnel, and hold the narrow opening up to your eye. When you look through the narrow end of the funnel, that's the world as you usually see it—going from a small tunnel to a widescreen view. Your world is wide, full of motion, and interesting. Now, turn the funnel around and look through the wide mouth. The perspective is flipped. That's the way someone with Alzheimer's views the world. It starts out big, then narrows to just that small opening. The peripheral things drop away, and those with Alzheimer's see—with laser focus—only what's right in front of them.

Learning about Alzheimer's, choosing to enter the world of a person with dementia, and adapting how you interact with your partner are wise steps for you to take. They give comfort to him or her, are necessary parts of coping, and help you as a caregiver survive. It is as your partner would choose it to be, as he or she would wish it to be. It is as you should choose it to be, as you should wish it to be.

Surviving Alzheimer's Disease

Life is good and I plan to have it continue that way until my children tell me it's time for a nursing home or something like that. This is realistic with what my Alzheimer's book says about my future. But 'til then, I will try my best to be normal—whatever that means—and keep my happy side of life always continuing. I'm lucky to have such a good family and many friends to help get me through all this. And so another great day to thank the Lord and smile, smile, smile.

— Elaine's notes during a visit to
Door County, Wisconsin, dated July 3, 2012

—CHAPTER 10—
Challenges

As a young state senator, I regularly heard one of the legislature's most bombastic orators. He was a legend in his own mind. He came from the western part of Wisconsin, along the Mississippi River. He bragged in his speeches about the "courage, fortitude, and conviction" of his constituents when dealing with the spring floodwaters of the mighty Mississippi.

Well, this silver-tongued senator passes away, and he's met at the pearly gates by St. Peter. "New arrivals have to give a speech," St. Peter says. The senator, with great confidence, tells St. Peter he will once again deliver his speech about the courage, fortitude, and conviction of his brave constituents as to how they met a flood along the Mississippi River in the springtime.

"That's well and good," says St. Peter, "but I want to warn you: Noah and his three sons will be in the audience."

* * *

Who am I to be talking about pain and hardship when you may be going through something much worse?

As challenges go, I'd like to think I've done all right. I accept the fact that I'm a work in progress. Not even Noah got everything right—he brought geese onboard, and we all know what a mess they can cause.

As I've climbed this mountain, I've succeeded in tiptoeing around some of the goose piles created by Alzheimer's and stepped smack dab into others. Maybe you can learn from my mistakes. My hope is that our discussion here can help you survive and be the best possible caregiver for your own situation.

What I wish I'd known

When your partner gets an Alzheimer's diagnosis, it's important to get started on a bucket list of things you want to experience together. Prioritizing helps you feel comfortable later on when you are alone and must do things without your spouse.

Elaine and I are ten years into this so-called journey. Some of the worst days are behind us.

I've received the phone call from my bewildered wife, lost while driving, surrounded by orange construction barrels, and trying to explain herself to a police officer. I've answered the same questions for her every five minutes. I've seen her confuse lipstick with nail polish and helped her when she couldn't figure out how to put on her bra. I've given away most of her clothes and her car.

None of that was pleasant.

But in so many ways, my cup runneth over.

We have terrific kids who love their parents very much. Even though our daughters live more than a thousand miles away, they visit often. All the kids come at the drop of a hat if I ask them or need them. Our grandchildren and great-grandchildren impress me with their talents and passions and inspire me to work toward a world without Alzheimer's for their generations.

We're blessed to live in a major urban area with access to great medical care and other resources that make a world of difference in Elaine's well-being, as well as mine.

I'm lucky enough to own a business. I can set my own hours and work from home. I can delegate responsibilities to a team I have trusted for years. When I require time off to devote to Elaine's needs, my business partners understand and cover for me so I don't have to worry about the day-to-day routine. Actually, the firm has done better without me and grown. I thank them for their great support and friendship.

If any of our employees are ever put into a caregiving situation—Alzheimer's-related or not—I'll have insights into the added challenges they are facing. I want to be understanding of their divided attention and give them the opportunity to carry out their responsibilities without worrying that their career will suffer.

I can only hope you are managing things. Nationwide, more than one-third of Alzheimer's caregivers reduce their hours at work or quit their jobs to provide care, losing an average of fifteen thousand dollars in annual income. How can they possibly absorb a financial hit like that? The Alzheimer's Association's 2016 Special Report provided some bleak answers: to make ends meet, one in five caregivers cuts back on his or her own doctor visits, and 11 percent don't get all of their own medications. The situation can be so dire that these heroes are 28 percent more likely to eat less or go hungry.

The report also talked about "care contributors," defined as people who at least once a month pay dementia-related expenses, provide care, or do both. These generous friends and family members spend more than five thousand dollars a year of their own money for groceries, medical supplies such as adult diapers, and in-home care. The price tag is many thousands more if the person with dementia lives in a care facility—maybe as much as one hundred thousand dollars a year. Many people assume that Medicare, Medicaid, or basic health insurance will cover nursing home costs, and sadly, that's just not the case. No wonder that 60 to 70 percent of people with Alzheimer's are cared for at home.

I know I am so, so fortunate in that I had purchased long-term care insurance (for both of us, in fact), which allowed Elaine to receive excellent daycare services for nearly four years and, now, allows her to be cared for in an outstanding assisted-living facility. Only 3 percent of American adults have such insurance. I'd like to think that being in that slim minority means I'm smart; in fact, this is the result of a principled, persistent, pestering, almost obnoxiously unbearable life insurance agent. (You know who you are, and I luv ya, kid!) That decision, years ago, has assured that Alzheimer's care won't bankrupt us.

So don't feel sorry for me.

My heart aches for you because you're just getting started. Your life's circumstances may be a lot more difficult than mine. Maybe you were struggling even before your spouse was diagnosed. Maybe your loved one has early-onset Alzheimer's, adding to the shock and sadness of your situation. Maybe you have health problems of your own. Maybe you don't have a good relationship with your children (or don't have children at all), so you lack that younger, more energetic supportive presence in your life. Maybe you live in a smaller community where the nearest adult day services program is an hour away. Maybe there are financial difficulties. Maybe it's some other misery or daily strain.

Any one of these challenges is reason to reach out—and I mean now—for help in surviving.

What I wish I'd done

I should have forgiven myself for not being perfect because I was doing the best I could in a difficult situation. It's understandable to have regrets about my shortcomings, but there is no point in feeling guilty.

If you ever hear of someone who is completely successful, healthy, and happy as an Alzheimer's caregiver by going it alone, let me know. That person should be written up in the medical journals and maybe even considered for sainthood.

I never realized how bad I had gotten until I overheard a phone conversation with whomever you were talking with on the phone, and I'm sorry to make life so difficult for us, and I guess I don't fully understand how difficult I've been for you. . . . I don't want to be a burden to you anymore. You deserve much more and I understand. And I want to thank you for all you have done for me and love you forever.

— A note from Elaine to Marty, date unknown

—CHAPTER 11—
What Surviving Looks Like

Years ago, I was flying early one morning on a business trip from Milwaukee to Washington, DC, and as I got on the plane, a very well-dressed, distinguished gentleman was speaking to the flight attendant. He was explaining to her that he needed her help because he had to get off the plane during its stopover in Detroit, and he was worried he might sleep through it. "Of course," the flight attendant said, "I'll make sure to wake you. I promise. I guarantee it."

To my surprise, as everyone got off the plane in Washington, who should I see but that well-dressed gentleman. His behavior was anything but distinguished— he was yelling and complaining at the flight attendant as he stormed away. I couldn't help but feel sorry for her.

"My goodness," I said, "that man was so angry."

She replied, "He's angry? You should have seen the fellow I put off the plane in Detroit."

* * *

Like that disgruntled passenger, when Alzheimer's entered your life, you were taken to a destination you did not choose. I didn't pick it either, but now that I have journeyed up that rocky mountain, I know where—and why—I made mistakes.

By now, I hope I've succeeded in telling you that in order to be a successful, loving caregiver, you need to first *learn* about the disease. Doing so makes it possible to *cope* with the heroics of caregiving. The third part of my mantra is *survive*.

I can be considered a survivor of Alzheimer's because it is a disease with two patients: the person with the diagnosis and the caregiver. I also use the word *survivor* because I anticipate I'll outlive Elaine. In a way, I already have. I am a widower with a wife.

As a survivor, I'm more sensitive to, and understanding of, what it means to lose someone you love. I'm more aware of other people's feelings, their challenges, their pain.

Survival is about peace of heart, knowing I've done all I could, including writing this book to hopefully help other caregivers. It also means I'm taking the time—and now I have the time—to be a better parent, a better grandparent, a better friend, and a better helper to others in this life. Once you've dealt with and adapted to the challenges of this dreaded disease, every role you play becomes more meaningful.

I survived the early stages of this disease when Elaine's behavior first pointed to trouble. I survived the transition from spouse to the ever-changing role of caregiver. I survived the heartache of watching the disease progress. Surprisingly, no one actually did punch me in the nose due to my irrational irritability.

In the middle stages of the disease, as I mentioned earlier, Elaine's sleep patterns made it impossible for me to get a decent night's rest. Sometimes, she'd be out of bed and wandering around the condo. She wasn't sure which door was to the bathroom and which one led outside. There's a busy street a block from our driveway, and Lake Michigan is just two blocks away. Knowing she could get lost in our home, I feared what she would do if she got outside. I had an extra lock put on the door, and I started sleeping on the couch. I hoped that, if Elaine did try to leave, I would hear her and could protect her from any harm.

At my age, night after night of poor sleep—in fact, year after year—took an insidious toll. My exhaustion and frustration became so severe that I had little left to give when the disease progressed to the late stages.

One day about eight years after Elaine's diagnosis, I was finishing a phone call with our daughter Kathy. "I love you," I said as I told her goodbye. Elaine overheard this and wanted to know whom was I talking with, so of course I told her it was our daughter Kathy. "We don't have a daughter named Kathy," she insisted. "Why would you make that up?" Her tone was most uncharacteristic, hostile and accusing. She insinuated that this Kathy had to be someone who was not to be associated with. "You've got to be up to no good," she said. She wanted to know whom else I was in love with. I knew it was the disease talking and not Elaine. She was the one who had told me that you can lose an election but you can't be defeated. This outburst, however, did defeat me. I began to seriously wonder, how much longer can I live with my wife, and how much longer can she live with me?

After loving Elaine for sixty-two years, I was angry with myself for even thinking this way.

* * *

I loved sailing from a young age. When we were in high school, I bought a rowboat, wanting to make it my very first sailboat. Elaine went to the Army Surplus Store and bought old parachute fabric that she fashioned into sails. As often happens, one boat led to another. Eventually, we owned real sailboats, one of which we named *True Love*, inspired by an old movie called *High Society*. In it, Bing Crosby sings a love song to Grace Kelly.

> *Suntanned, windblown*
> *Honeymooners at last alone*
> *Feeling far above par*
> *Oh, how lucky we are*

While I give to you and you give to me
True love, true love
So on and on it will always be
True love, true love

Six months a year, we'd be out on the waters off Milwaukee and, farther north in Wisconsin, off the Door County peninsula. On a sailboat, you're in the elements, which is fun when you're young and romantic, and you go where the wind takes you. What great times! As the years went by, we traded the labor of sailing a boat for a forty-six-foot cruising trawler that we named *Beyond Ayes* because it represented a life beyond anything I thought I would ever have.

We had the adventure of a lifetime on that trawler with our friends Judy and Ron—a five-thousand-mile trip we did in segments from 2005 through 2007. On a route called "America's Great Loop," we rode the current through Illinois and south on the Ohio River and the Tombigbee Waterway to Mobile, Alabama. From there, it was around Florida, and then we motored up the Eastern Seaboard at seven knots to the Hudson River, the Erie Canal, the Great Lakes, and home again. We shared the Mississippi River with barges full of coal and passed by the Statue of Liberty. We celebrated the success of my cancer treatments, and we ate well and laughed so much. But even then, uncertainty was creeping in when Elaine did some strange things, like putting the salt and pepper shakers "away" in the oven. Little did we realize that the odd behaviors actually were early symptoms of Alzheimer's.

Our boat has been our second home. Over Memorial Day weekend 2015, the four of us went out on the water together for what proved to be the last time.

I was hoping the long holiday weekend on the boat would be just as enjoyable as the Great Loop trip a decade earlier. I could catch up with Judy and Ron, and they could help keep an eye on Elaine. But, even in that small space, Elaine got lost. In the middle of the night, Ron woke me to say Elaine had come to their tiny sleeping quarters, asking, "Where is Marty?" She'd had to climb over me to leave our bed! I'll never know what possessed her to do that, and I shudder to think what would have happened had she gone out onto the deck. That told me just how rapidly the disease was progressing. I could never leave her alone. Never. It was time for Elaine to live elsewhere. Yet, I still felt guilt.

My counselor at the Alzheimer's Association had opened the conversation a year earlier. "When the time comes," she said, "you are not 'putting' her in a nursing home. You are not 'putting' her anyplace. Her illness is causing her to have more needs than one person can handle, even with adult daycare and in-home help. You cannot respond to all of her needs. A dementia care unit can, with trained staff who are new and fresh every eight hours. You will be giving her an opportunity to be at the best place she could be."

She wasn't the only one suggesting a move for Elaine. Many others had been asking why Elaine was still living at home. That's the toughest question a caregiver has to face—ironically, sometimes it comes from the very people who doubted the Alzheimer's diagnosis in the first place. But you know me: I'm stubborn.

Moving to a facility was never going to cure Elaine. I knew that. But I also recognized that Marty's One-Man Nursing Home no longer was good enough either. That realization made it somewhat easier for me to accept the inevitable: Elaine should move. After all, to quote a seventeenth-century poem I read in high school, "stone walls do not a prison make."

Our children and I did some research, taking tours of care facilities and asking a lot of questions. We watched to see how attentive the staff was and whether the residents seemed interested in the activities that were offered. We were lucky to have options, including the two facilities where Elaine had most recently attended day programs. After weighing the pros and cons of the facilities, we made arrangements for Elaine to move to the residential memory unit of the same place where she first attended a day program.

None of that made it any easier when The Day came.

It was horrible to take her there. As we left our home, she accidentally left the door open as she followed me out into the attached garage. I didn't have the heart to tell her to close the door behind her because it marked the end of that life as we knew it. Instead of taking her to the adult daycare center where she'd gone five days a week for the previous two years, we drove ten miles to her new home. It is a caring, compassionate place. She deserves nothing less. Her room is comfortable but small with the intent that she spend most of her day with other residents and in activities. In advance, we had hung family photos in hopes of giving her touchstones to her past.

The facility's staff advised me to avoid visiting for the first five days, so that Elaine could become acclimated. It was so difficult to be separated from her, but I had to trust that it was best for her. We did talk on the phone a couple times. They showed her a short video I had recorded in which I told her I was busy in Madison and would see her soon. A bit of therapeutic fibbing.

Even as I adjusted to the emptiness in my home and in my heart, there were two emotions dominating my thinking: relief that Elaine would be safe and hope that now I could focus on being a better father and grandfather. It was like competing in a relay race. You run your hardest, and then you hand off the baton to someone with strong, untired legs. Let's face it, you're never going to find someone who says, "Hooray for me! I put my wife in a nursing home!" But I do know this: we both are in a better place. I now get a better night's sleep. I get my exercise. I have a better chance of being healthy. And I no longer worry every minute about Elaine.

I visit her almost every day, and I am learning to not feel guilty when I don't. She deserves my best attention, and she picks up on it if I'm preoccupied. When I'm over-stressed, I'm better off—and more importantly, she's better off—if I stay away.

As a person with late-stage Alzheimer's, there is a silver lining in this very dark cloud that envelops Elaine. It's that she lacks awareness of all she's lost: her independence, her memories, her future. She is not upset by the fact that she lives in a care facility and wears an adult diaper. And, because she no longer is anxious, neither am I.

The less she knows me, the less she demands of me. It is my hope that she is experiencing a familiar voice, one that makes her feel comforted. I make a point to tell her what a wonderful wife, mother, and grandmother she is. I thank her for all she's done for me.

We still enjoy car rides and dining out. We are limited only by my imagination and energy. When we walk around the shopping mall near her care facility, we see lots of young children. In those moments, she hands out compliments as readily as she did at the Executive

Residence or in her preschool classroom. "You're a cutie," she'll say. *That's* my Elaine.

I'm getting ready for a move, too—back to sleeping in a bed. Even after Elaine went into assisted living, I've still felt her presence so strongly in our bedroom that I've continued for almost a year to sleep on the couch. I've now decided to make a clean break from some of the bad memories by moving into a smaller, ground-floor condo in our complex. No more stairs is a good thing for someone who's had the health problems I've had.

Home, I've learned, isn't a building. It's a place inside you where you feel secure. That goes for both of us.

Elaine's new place of residence is across town from me. She has left our condo behind for good. Now, she lives just a couple of miles from Milwaukee Lutheran High School, where we spent our first years together. In a way, we've come full circle.

I am so very lucky I met Miss Elaine Ruth Thaney in freshman Latin class, lucky to have her fall in love with me, lucky she said yes, lucky she supported every dream and crazy idea I ever had, lucky she raised such great kids, lucky I still get to hold her hand every day. If Alzheimer's is the worst thing that can happen to me, I've got the best of the worst.

If Alzheimer's Could Speak

By Tara Reed

Talk to me . . .
I can hear your words and they still touch my soul.

Smile at me . . .
My eyes can see you and feel your heart
even if I don't remember how to smile back.

Hold my hand . . .
I can feel your energy when our hands connect.
It makes me feel safe and less alone.

Love me . . .
My heart can feel your love even if
my words can't express mine.

Live your life . . .
Help me on my path but don't press pause
on your life. Be the vibrant person I know & love.

Trust the process . . .
I know this is hard and not what we planned
but trust the process. We can't control it but
we can choose our focus. Remember the good
times, know that I am OK and that you are in my
heart always.

Acknowledgments

The authors are grateful to their families for their support, encouragement, and invaluable contributions during this project. Marty particularly thanks his children Kathy, Marty, Kristine, and Matt, as well as Bob and Rose Schreiber, Jill Schreiber, and Bill and Marion Schreiber. Cathy thanks her husband Kent Lowry and daughter Greta.

Marty also thanks his business partners at Martin Schreiber & Associates, Inc., for their extraordinary patience and friendship and gives special thanks to Denise Cifaldi for helping in countless ways. We know that writing this book took longer than we told you it would, so thanks for hanging in there.

Thank you also to Lynda Markut, education and support coordinator; MaryAnn Vance, development director; and the entire staff of the Southeastern Wisconsin Chapter of the Alzheimer's Association. They cheered us on every step of the way.

Many others helped by editing the manuscript without destroying our spirits, including Judy Banta, Betsy Benson, Bill Christofferson, David Cross, Hugh and Mary Denison, Jim Haney, Al and Anne Iding, Tom Krajewski, Lynn Krebs, Fred and Colleen Latzke, Stephanie Leanes, Ron and Judy Lokken, Anita and Bob Pietrykowski, Kate Huston Raab, Sue Schalk, Bob Schulze, Pete Schumacher, Don and Karen Six, Ann Stacy, Edie Starrett, Tom and Sue Thaney, John Vitek, Ralph Weber, and Maria Welk.

We also honor the memory of Kitty Rhoades, secretary of the Wisconsin Department of Health Services. Kitty was committed to ensuring all that she served had a voice, especially those suffering from dementia, mental illness, and disabilities.

In addition, Marty thanks caregivers he has met and the authors of the many Alzheimer's-related books. Your insights are making a big difference in people's lives.

Cathy honors family members who have suffered from dementia, including Anna McClintock, Ralph Breitenbucher, Karl McClintock, and Helen Farrar. The loving example provided by their caregivers through the past forty years has been an inspiration.

Resources

Alzheimer's Association
- national 24/7 helpline (1-800-272-3900)
- alz.org

You also can follow the association on Facebook, Twitter, YouTube, Google+, Pinterest, and Instagram.

Other resources may be available in your area, sponsored by the county, state, or federal government. Services they provide may include:
- information about options for long-term care
- elder abuse and crisis intervention
- information about public and private benefits
- community-based services
- home-delivered meals
- caregiver respite
- transportation

Look for organizations with names such as:
- Aging and Disability Resource Center

- Aging Resource Center
- Area Agency on Aging
- County Department on Aging

You can research nursing homes in your area at: medicare. gov/nursinghomecompare. Facilities are given one to five stars as an overall rating, as well as for health inspections, staffing levels, and how well the facility cares for its residents' needs.

About the Authors

Martin J. Schreiber grew up in Milwaukee. Inspired by his father's example as a member of the Wisconsin State Assembly and the Milwaukee City Council, Martin ran for public office even before he had completed law school. In 1962, he was elected as the youngest-ever member of the Wisconsin State Senate. He was elected lieutenant governor in 1970 and, in 1977, became the thirty-ninth governor of Wisconsin. Today, he heads a public affairs firm in Milwaukee and is an advocate for Alzheimer's caregivers. He and his wife Elaine are the parents of four children: Kathryn Lyon, Marty Schreiber, Kristine Haas, and Matt Schreiber. They have thirteen grandchildren and five great-grandchildren.

Cathy Breitenbucher is a Milwaukee-based writer who can trace her interest in medicine to dinner-table conversations with her parents, a nurse and a laboratory technician. She is a native Iowan and graduate of the University of Iowa. She had a thirteen-year career as a full-time newspaper sportswriter, highlighted by covering the Olympic Games in 1984 and 1988. Since 1992, she has been a freelance writer for publications such as People magazine, *USA Today*, the *Washington Post*, and several Milwaukee-area magazines and newspapers. This is her third book. She is married and has one daughter.